T0184834

Data Analysis in Medicine and Health Using R

In medicine and health, data are analyzed to guide treatment plans, patient care and control and prevention policies. However, in doing so, researchers in medicine and health often lack the understanding of data and statistical concepts and the skills in programming. In addition, there is also an increasing demand for data analyses to be reproducible, along with more complex data that require cutting-edge analysis. This book provides readers with both the fundamental concepts of data and statistical analysis and modeling. It also has the skills to perform the analysis using the R programming language, which is the lingua franca for statisticians. The topics in the book are presented in a sequence to minimize the time to help readers understand the objectives of data and statistical analysis, learn the concepts of statistical modeling and acquire the skills to perform the analysis. The R codes and datasets used in the book will be made available on GitHub for easy access. The book will also be live on the website bookdown.org, a service provided by RStudio, PBC, to host books written using the bookdown package in the R programming language.

Analytics and AI for Healthcare

Series Editor: Nilmini Wickramasinghe, Swinburne University of Technology

About the Series
Artificial Intelligence (AI) and analytics are increasingly being applied to various health-care settings. AI and analytics are salient to facilitate better understanding and identifying key insights from healthcare data in many areas of practice and enquiry in healthcare in-cluding at the genomic, individual, hospital, community and/or population levels.

The Chapman & Hall/CRC Press Analytics and AI in Healthcare Series aims to help pro-fessionals upskill and leverage the techniques, tools, technologies and tactics of analytics and AI to achieve better healthcare delivery, access and outcomes.

The series covers all areas of analytics and AI as applied to healthcare. It will look at critical areas, including prevention, prediction, diagnosis, treatment, monitoring, rehabilitation and survivorship.

Explainable Artificial Intelligence in Healthcare: Unboxing Machine Learning in Pre-pro-cessing and Medical Imaging
Edited by Mehul S Raval, Mohendra Roy, Tolga Kaya, and Rupal Kapdi

Data Analysis in Medicine and Health Using R
Kamarul Imran Musa, Wan Nor Arifin Wan Mansor, and Tengku Muhammad Hanis

For more information about this series please visit: https://www.routledge.com/analytics-and-ai-for-healthcare/book-series/Aforhealth

Data Analysis in Medicine and Health Using R

Kamarul Imran Musa
Wan Nor Arifin Wan Mansor
Tengku Muhammad Hanis

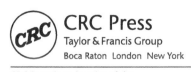

CRC Press
Taylor & Francis Group
Boca Raton London New York

CRC Press is an imprint of the
Taylor & Francis Group, an **informa** business

A CHAPMAN & HALL BOOK

First edition published 2024
by CRC Press
6000 Broken Sound Parkway NW, Suite 300, Boca Raton, FL 33487-2742

and by CRC Press
4 Park Square, Milton Park, Abingdon, Oxon, OX14 4RN

CRC Press is an imprint of Taylor & Francis Group, LLC

© 2024 Kamarul Imran Musa, Wan Nor Arifin Wan Mansor, and Tengku Muhammad Hanis

Reasonable efforts have been made to publish reliable data and information, but the author and publisher cannot assume responsibility for the validity of all materials or the consequences of their use. The authors and publishers have attempted to trace the copyright holders of all material reproduced in this publication and apologize to copyright holders if permission to publish in this form has not been obtained. If any copyright material has not been acknowledged please write and let us know so we may rectify in any future reprint.

Except as permitted under U.S. Copyright Law, no part of this book may be reprinted, reproduced, transmitted, or utilized in any form by any electronic, mechanical, or other means, now known or hereafter invented, including photocopying, microfilming, and recording, or in any information storage or retrieval system, without written permission from the publishers.

For permission to photocopy or use material electronically from this work, access www.copyright. com or contact the Copyright Clearance Center, Inc. (CCC), 222 Rosewood Drive, Danvers, MA 01923, 978-750-8400. For works that are not available on CCC please contact mpkbookspermissions@tandf.co.uk

Trademark notice: Product or corporate names may be trademarks or registered trademarks and are used only for identification and explanation without intent to infringe.

ISBN: 978-1-032-28415-6 (hbk)
ISBN: 978-1-032-28414-9 (pbk)
ISBN: 978-1-003-29677-5 (ebk)

DOI: 10.1201/9781003296775

Typeset in Alegreya font
by KnowledgeWorks Global Ltd

Publisher's note: This book has been prepared from camera-ready copy provided by the authors.

Kamarul Imran Musa (KIM) would like to dedicate this book to his parents (Arwah Hj Musa and Napisah Mohamed Nor) and his parents-in-law, his wife (Juhara Haron), his sons (Afif and Iman) and to all his students.

Wan Nor Arifin Wan Mansor (WNA) would like to dedicate this book to researchers in medicine, public health and health sciences who are brave enough to learn R. You are the heroes of the future!

Tengku Muhammad Hanis would like to dedicate this book to his parents (Tengku Mokhtar and Nor Malaysia), his wife (Nurul Asmaq) and all his fantastic teachers and lecturers.

Contents

Preface

We wrote this book to help new R programming users with limited programming and statistical backgrounds. We understand the struggles they are going through to move from point-and-click statistical software such as SPSS or MS Excel to more code-centric software such as R and Python. From our experiences, frustration sets in early in learning this code-centric software. It often demotivates new users to the extent that they ditch them and return to using point-and-click statistical software. This book will minimize these struggles and gently help these excited but fragile new users to learn quickly and effectively the codes and workflows to perform data and statistical analysis using the R programming language.

This book's audience includes postgraduate students, public health researchers, epidemiologists and biostatisticians. We designed and wrote this book based on our experiences teaching students in the public health, epidemiology and biostatistics programs at the School of Medical Sciences, Universiti Sains Malaysia. Between KIM and WNA, we have over 30 years of experience teaching and training undergraduate and postgraduate students. As we mentioned earlier, most of our postgraduate students are students in the public health, epidemiology or biostatistics programs at the School of Medical Sciences, Universiti Sains Malaysia.

The courses we teach include basic and advanced statistics, multivariable data analysis, structural equation modeling, advanced numerical data analysis and advanced categorical data analysis. This book, we believe, will achieve its objective. The main objective is to help new R programming users (such as our undergraduate and postgraduate students) quickly understand the R programming language, make plots, explore data, summarize data and perform statistical analyses inside RStudio IDE. We also provide the interpretation of graphs, tables and statistical models relevant to our students and us. They do not have strong mathematical and statistical backgrounds; however, in their career, they are very much involved with collecting, analyzing and interpreting data. Some will work at medical and health institutions and organizations. Their applied knowledge and skills in data analysis and epidemiological and statistical models will help them draw health policies and make evidence-based public health interventions.

We used the **rmarkdown** package[1] and the **bookdown** package[2] to write this book inside RStudio IDE. We are truly grateful to all the people who have developed both

---

[1]https://rmarkdown.rstudio.com/
[2]https://github.com/rstudio/bookdown

packages and to Posit Software[3]. Posit Software PBC is an Open Source Data Science Company, previously known as RStudio PBC. Posit Software PBC continuously supports open-source data science initiatives and develops and distributes the fantastic RStudio IDE[4]. When writing this physical book, we used R version 4.2.2 and RStudio version 2022.07.2 Build 576.

The source codes for the book are available on our GitHub repository[5] and also provided the datasets in the **data** folder at GitHub[6]. We are indebted to George Knott, the statistics editor at Chapman & Hall (CRC Press), who has been very supportive and understanding when we are chasing the datelines of the book. We also appreciate the help of Nivedita Menon, who has taken over the publishing task from George after he moved from his role at Chapman & Hall (CRC Press). In addition, Chapman & Hall (CRC Press) has been very kind to allow us to have the online version of the book on the bookdown website[7]. All in all, we hope everyone enjoys this book!

Kamarul Imran Musa[8]

Wan Nor Arifin Wan Mansor[9]

Tengku Muhammad Hanis[10]

School of Medical Sciences,
Universiti Sains Malaysia
2023-04-22

---

[3]https://posit.co/
[4]https://posit.co/products/open-source/rstudio/
[5]https://github.com/drkamarul/multivar_data_analysis
[6]https://github.com/drkamarul/multivar_data_analysis/tree/main/data
[7]https://bookdown.org/drki_musa/dataanalysis/
[8]https://github.com/drkamarul
[9]https://github.com/wnarifin
[10]https://github.com/tengku-hanis

1

R, RStudio and RStudio Cloud

1.1 Objectives

At the end of the chapter, the readers will

- be introduced to the R programming language
- be introduced to RStudio IDE
- be introduced to RStudio Cloud. RStudio Cloud is a platform where users can run RStudio on the cloud
- be able to install R on their local machine
- be able to install RStudio IDE on their local machine
- understand how to install LaTeX editor (Miktex or Tex Live and MacTex). A LaTeX editor is optional but is required if users want to render PDF outputs
- understand the structure of R scripts work
- understand R packages and R Taskview

1.2 Introduction

R is a language and environment for statistical computing and graphics. It is a GNU project similar to the S language and environment developed at Bell Laboratories. R provides a wide variety of statistical (linear and nonlinear modeling, classical statistical tests, time-series analysis, classification, clustering and others) and graphical techniques and is highly extensible.

One of R's strengths is the ease with which well-designed publication-quality plots can be produced, including mathematical symbols and formulae where needed. R is available as Free Software under the terms of the Free Software Foundation's GNU General Public License in source code form. It compiles and runs on various UNIX platforms and similar systems (including FreeBSD and Linux), Windows and macOS.

DOI: 10.1201/9781003296775-1

1

1.3   RStudio IDE

RStudio is an integrated development environment (IDE) for R. It includes a console and syntax-highlighting editor that supports direct code execution and tools for plotting, history, debugging and workspace management.

RStudio is available in open source and commercial editions and runs on the desktop (Windows, Mac, and Linux) or in a browser connected to RStudio Server or RStudio Workbench (Debian/Ubuntu, Red Hat/CentOS and SUSE Linux).

1.4   RStudio Cloud

RStudio Cloud by RStudio facilitates the learning of R. Anyone can sign up and start using RStudio on the cloud. It is one of the quickest ways to learn R.

Using RStudio Cloud, we do not have to install R on our local machine. RStudio Cloud allows collaboration between R teachers and students. It also helps colleagues work together on R projects.

RStudio described it as a lightweight, cloud-based solution that allows anyone to do, share, teach and learn data science online. And it also adds that by using this platform, we can

- analyze our data using the RStudio IDE directly from our browser
- share projects with our team, class, workshop or the world
- teach data science with R to our students or colleagues
- learn data science in an instructor-led environment or with interactive tutorials

RStudio Cloud has the free and the commercial version (which is fortunately very affordable). To start using RStudio Cloud, visit https://rstudio.cloud/. On the page, click 'Sign Up'.

With RStudio Cloud, there is almost nothing to configure and you do not need dedicated hardware, installation or annual purchase contract required. Individual users, instructors and students only need a browser to do, share, teach and learn data science.

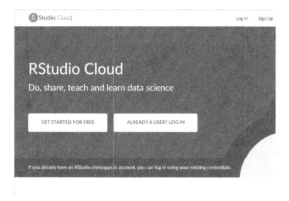

FIGURE 1.1
Sign up page for RStudio Cloud.

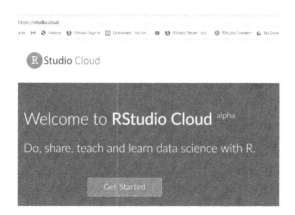

FIGURE 1.2
RStudio Cloud webpage.

1.4.1 The RStudio Cloud registration

This is the registration and login webpage for RStudio Cloud.

1.4.2 Register and log in

Proceed with registration. If you have Google account or GitHub account, you can use either one to quickly register. After you complete the registration, you can log into RStudio Cloud.

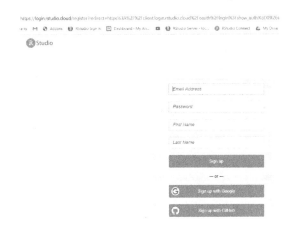

FIGURE 1.3
RStudio Cloud registration page.

1.5   Point and Click Graphical User Interface (GUI)

There are a number of GUI versions of R, also known as R GUI. The interface resembles a popular statistical software SPSS. For example, there are

- Bluesky statistics https://www.blueskystatistics.com/
- jamovi https://www.jamovi.org/

BlueSky Statistics can help users to

- migrate from expensive propriety statistical applications to R
- ease the R learning curve
- use the cutting-edge analytics available in R without having to learn programming
- get results in true word processing tables automatically
- quickly add your own menus and dialog boxes to any R functions

And this is **jamovi** software. jamovi aims to be a neutral platform and takes no position with respect to competing statistical philosophies. The project was not founded to promote a particular statistical ideology, instead wanting to serve as a safe space where different statistical approaches might be published side-by-side and consider themselves first-rate members of the jamovi community.

jamovi is an interesting software. It is a new 'third generation' statistical spreadsheet. It is designed from the ground up to be easy to use, it is a compelling alternative to costly statistical products such as SPSS and SAS. jamovi is built on top of the R statistical language, giving you access to the best the statistics community has to

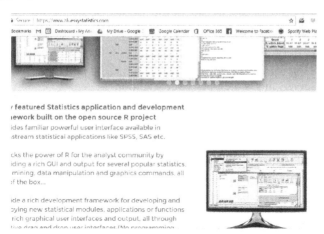

featured Statistics application and development
ework built on the open source R project
ides familiar powerful user interface available in
stream statistical applications like SPSS, SAS etc.

cks the power of R for the analyst community by
iding a rich GUI and output for several popular statistics,
mining, data manipulation and graphics commands, all
f the box...

ide a rich development framework for developing and
oying new statistical modules, applications or functions
rich graphical user interfaces and output, all through

FIGURE 1.4
Bluesky statistics software interface.

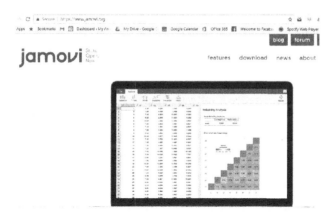

FIGURE 1.5
jamovi software.

offer. jamovi will always be free and open because jamovi is made by the scientific community, for the scientific community.

1.6 RStudio Server

You can run R and RStudio on the server. To do this you have to install RStudio Workbench. Previously, R Studio Workbench was known as RStudio Server.

By using RStudio Server, R users can perform analysis on the server. Using RStudio server can give you a taste of cloud data analysis.

There are two versions of RStudio server:

- RStudio Server: This is the Open Source edition
- RStudio Workbench: This is the Professional edition

At our medical school. we have RStudio Server Professional Edition (**courtesy of** RStudio, of course) running on our server here https://healthdata.usm.my/rstudio/auth-sign-in

---

1.7   Installing R and RStudio on Your Local Machine

To install R on your local machine, you have to have **Admin Right** to your machine. We recommend that you install

- **R** first,
- then **RStudio**

1.7.1   Installing R

Though you can use the native R software (that you just installed) to run R codes, we highly encourage you to use RStudio Integrated Desktop Environment (IDE).

We will show this step by step. First, let us install R on your machine. To install R, go to cran[1]. Then choose the R version that's correct for your machine OS. For example, for Windows OS, the link is https://cran.r-project.org/bin/windows/base/R-4.3.1-win.exe. And for Mac OS, the download link is https://cran.r-project.org/bin/macosx/big-sur-x86_64/base/R-4.3.1-x86_64.pkg. Similarly, if you are using Linux, follow the steps as listed before.

It is always recommended that users install the latest version of R. During this writing, the latest version is R version 4.2.1 known as Funny-Looking Kid version that was released on June 23, 2022. Users can have multiple R versions on the same local machines. So you do not need to uninstall the old R version to install a new R version.

1.7.2   Installing RStudio IDE

Now, to install RStudio IDE, go to the RStudio download[2] page. Choose the supported platforms correct for your machine OS. The size of the download will be around 90–110 MB.

---

[1]https://cran.r-project.org/
[2]https://www.rstudio.com/products/rstudio/download/#download

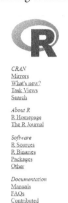
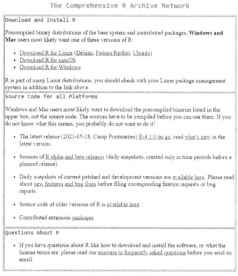

FIGURE 1.6
CRAN website.

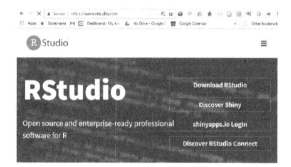

FIGURE 1.7
RStudio website.

1.7.3 Checking R and RStudio installations

Now, we assume you have installed both R and RStudio. To make sure they work perfectly (or at least for the first time), check:

- Does your machine can load R? Depending on your OS, go and start R.

- What version of R do you have? When R loads, look for the version of R.

- Do you have RStudio? Depending on your OS, go and start RStudio.

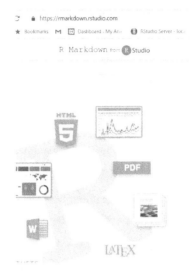

FIGURE 1.8
R Markdown.

- What version of RStudio do you have? When RStudio loads, look for the version of R. If you have multiple R version, you can choose the R version of your choice by going to **Tools** then **Global Options** then **General**.

- Do you need to update R and RStudio? By knowing the versions of R and RStudio, now you know if you need to update both or one of them.

1.7.4   TinyTeX, MiKTeX or MacTeX (for Mac OS) and TeX live

Based on experience, as R users develop more R skills, they may find converting their analysis into PDF documents desirable. It is necessary to install a LaTeX editor if they want to convert the outputs they generated in R into PDF format. However, if they do not need to produce a PDF document, they do not have to install it. If they require more flexibility to edit their LaTeX codes, then they may think of getting common LaTeX editors such as MiKtex, MacTeX or TeX Live.

We encourage users to first install TinyTeX. If you render your R document into PDF just by using TinyTeX, then that's enough. To install TinyTeX, follow the instruction from https://yihui.org/tinytex/ . For R users, it is simple running these two codes `install.packages('tinytex')` and `tinytex::install_tinytex()`

Install **MiKTeX** as your LaTeX editor if your machine is using Window OS. If you use MacOS, then install **MacTeX**.

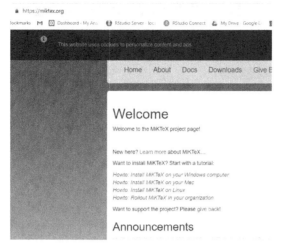

FIGURE 1.9
MikTeX webpage.

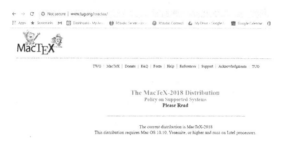

FIGURE 1.10
MacTeX webpage.

1.8 Starting Your RStudio

You can either login to RStudio Cloud and automatically see the RStudio interface OR you can start RStudio on your local machine by loading it. Remember, to login to RStudio Cloud, go to https://rstudio.cloud. You will be asked for your username and password.

Click this link[3]

To start R on your machine, and if you are using Windows, find the RStudio program in your start bar on your machine. And start it. You will see an interface like the one

---

[3]https://rstudio.cloud/spaces/156361/join?access_code=WtlSxNuTm%2Fz7E%2BLb%2FW2XnOw48O%2BBTmL4B%2FqjYRIg

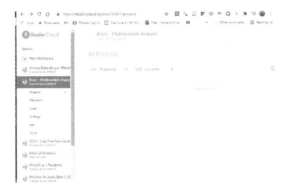

FIGURE 1.11
RStudio Cloud space for this book.

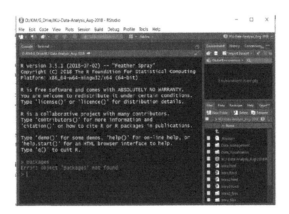

FIGURE 1.12
Rstudio Interface with Vibrant Ink theme.

below. This interface differs from what you see on your screen because I use the Vibrant Ink Theme. To choose the theme of your choice, click Global Options, then click Appearance. There are several themes available for you to choose.

What you see on RStudio now? You should see three panes if you start RStudio for the first time or four panes if you have used RStudio before.

1.8.1   Console tab

In Console tab, this is where we will see most of the results generated from codes in RStudio.

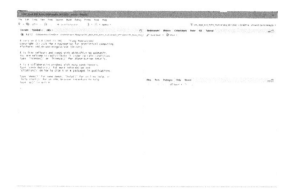

FIGURE 1.13
RStudio Panes.

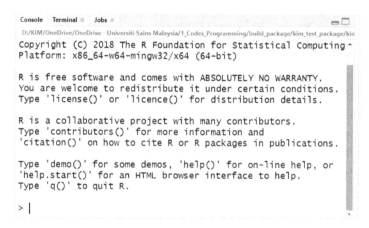

FIGURE 1.14
Console tab.

1.8.2   Files, plots, packages, help and viewer pane

In this console, you will see

- List of objects (Remember, R is an object-oriented-programming or **oop**)
- R files, datasets, tables, list, etc.

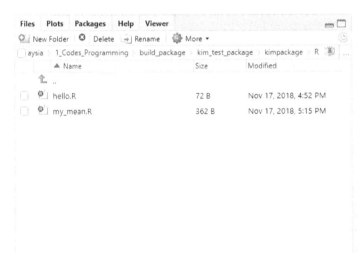

FIGURE 1.15
File, Plots, Packages, Help and Viewer pane.

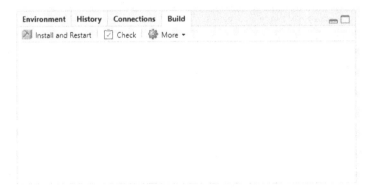

FIGURE 1.16
Environment, History, Connections and Build pane.

1.8.3   Environment, history, connection and build pane

In the environment, history, connection and build pane, you will see this

1.8.4   Source pane

In the Source pane, you can create R files and write your R codes

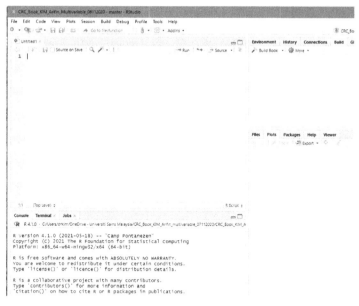

FIGURE 1.17
Source pane.

1.9 Summary

In this chapter, we learn about R, RStudio IDE and RStudio Cloud. We have also introduced two point and click R GUIs Bluesky Statistics and jamovi. To use RStudio without any hassle during installation, we recommend using RStudio Cloud.

2

R Scripts and R Packages

2.1 Objectives

At the end of this chapter, readers will be able

- to write simple R scripts
- to understand R packages
- to install R packages
- to create a new RStudio project
- to be able to use RStudio Cloud

2.2 Introduction

An R script is simply **a text file containing (almost) the same commands that you would enter on the command line of R**. (almost) refers to the fact that if you are using sink() to send the output to a file, you will have to enclose some commands in print() to get the same output as on the command line.

R packages are **extensions to the R statistical programming language**. R packages contain code, data and documentation in a standardized collection format that can be installed by users of R, typically via a centralized software repository such as CRAN (the Comprehensive R Archive Network).

2.3 Open a New Script

For beginners, you may start by writing some simple codes. Since these codes are written in R language, we call these codes as R scripts. To do this, go to **File**, then click **R Script**

- File -> R Script
- In Window OS, users can use this shortcut CTRL-SHIFT-N

DOI: 10.1201/9781003296775-2

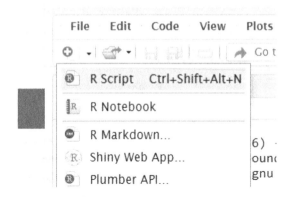

FIGURE 2.1
New R script.

2.3.1 Our first R script

Let us write our very first R codes inside an R script.

- In Line 1, type 2 + 3
- click CTRL-ENTER or CMD-ENTER
- see the outputs in the Console Pane

```
2 + 3
```

```
## [1] 5
```

After writing your codes inside the R script, you can save the R script file. This will allow you to open it up again to continue your work.

And to save R script, go to

- File ->
- Save As ->
- Choose folder ->

- Name the file

Now, types these codes to check the version of your R software

```
version[6:7]
```

```
##            _
## status
## major   4
```

The current version for R is 4.2.1

By they way if you are using lower version of R, then we recommend you to upgrade. To upgrade your R software

- and if you are using Windows, you can use **installr** package
- but if you use macOS, you may need to download R again and manually install

You may find more information from this link[1].

2.3.2 Function, argument and parameters

R codes contain

- function
- argument
- parameters

```
f <- function(<arguments>) {
## Do something interesting
}
```

For example, to list all the arguments for a function, you may use args(). Let's examine the arguments for the function lm(), a function to estimate parameters for linear regression model.

```
args(lm)
```

```
## function (formula, data, subset, weights, na.action, method = "qr",
##     model = TRUE, x = FALSE, y = FALSE, qr = TRUE, singular.ok = TRUE,
##     contrasts = NULL, offset, ...)
## NULL
```

Once you understand the required arguments, you may use the parameters so the function can perform the desired task. For example:

```
lm(weight ~ Time, data = ChickWeight)
```

```
##
## Call:
## lm(formula = weight ~ Time, data = ChickWeight)
##
## Coefficients:
## (Intercept)         Time
##      27.467        8.803
```

[1]https://www.linkedin.com/pulse/3-methods-update-r-rstudio-windows-mac-woratana-ngarmtrakulchol/

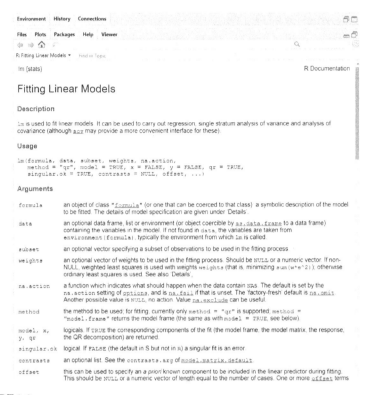

FIGURE 2.2

Help pane.

2.3.3   If users require further help

If users would like to see more extensive guides on certain functions, they may type the ? before the function. For example, if users want to know more about the function lm, then they may type the R codes below. Following that, R will open a help page with a more detailed description, usage of the function and the relevant arguments.

```
?lm
```

```
## starting httpd help server ... done
```

Here, we provide an example how a Help Pane will look like.

2.4   Packages

R is a programming language. Furthermore, R software runs on packages. R packages are collections of functions and data sets developed by the community. They

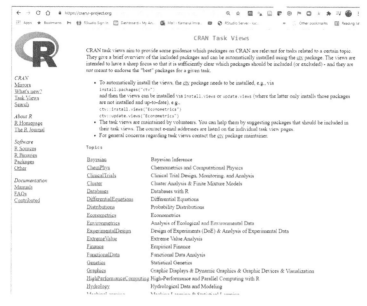

FIGURE 2.3
CRAN task views.

increase the power of R by improving existing base R codes and functions or by adding new ones.

A package is a suitable way to organize users' work and share it with others if users want to. Typically, a package will include

- code (sometimes not just R codes but codes in other programming languages),
- documentation for the package and the functions inside,
- some tests to check that everything works as it should, and
- data sets.

Users can read more about R packages here[2].

2.4.1 Packages on CRAN

At the time of writing, the CRAN package repository features 12784 packages. Available R packages are listed on the Cran Task Views website.

CRAN task views aim to provide some guidance which packages on CRAN are relevant for tasks related to a certain topic. They give a brief overview of the included packages and can be automatically installed using the **ctv** package.

---

[2]https://www.datacamp.com/community/tutorials/r-packages-guide

The views are intended to have a sharp focus so that it is sufficiently clear which packages should be included (or excluded), and they are not meant to endorse the "best" packages for a given task.

2.4.2   Checking availability of R package

To check if the desired package is available on users' machine, users can this inside their R console:

```
library(tidyverse)
```

```
## -- Attaching core tidyverse packages ----------------------- tidyverse 2.0.0 -
-
## v dplyr      1.1.1      v readr      2.1.4
## v forcats    1.0.0      v stringr    1.5.0
## v ggplot2    3.4.2      v tibble     3.2.1
## v lubridate  1.9.2      v tidyr      1.3.0
## v purrr      1.0.1
##          --        Conflicts       ----------------------------------------
tidyverse_conflicts() --
## x dplyr::filter() masks stats::filter()
## x dplyr::lag()    masks stats::lag()
##      i    Use    the    conflicted    package    (<http://conflicted.r-
lib.org/>) to force all conflicts to become errors
```

Users should not receive any error messages. Users who have not installed the package will receive an error message. Furthermore, it tells them that the package is not available in their R. By default, the package is stored in the R folder in their My Document or HOME directory

```
.libPaths()
```

```
## [1] "C:/Users/drkim/AppData/Local/R/win-library/4.2"
## [2] "C:/Program Files/R/R-4.2.3/library"
```

2.4.3   Install an R package

To install an R package, there are two ways:

   1.   users can type the R codes like below (without the # tag)

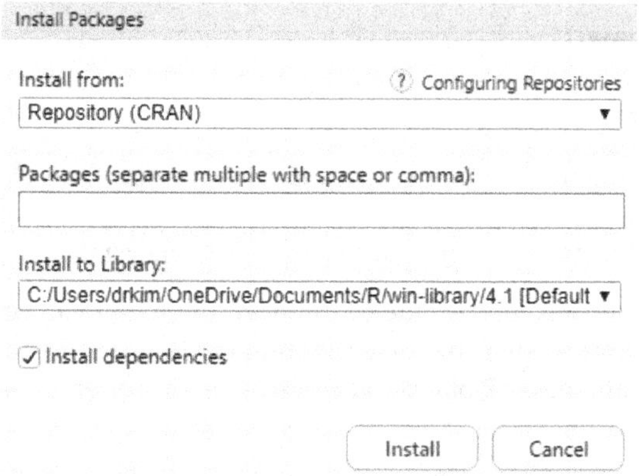

FIGURE 2.4
Install packages pane.

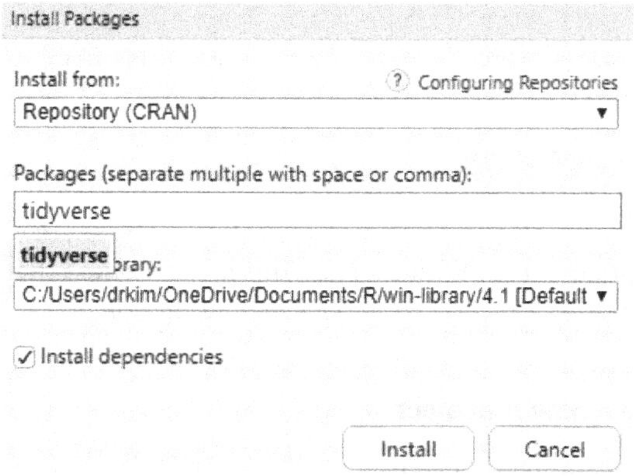

FIGURE 2.5
The name of the package to be installed.

```
# install.packages(tidyverse, dependencies = TRUE)
```

2. users can use the GUI in the RStudio IDE

Now, type the package you want to install. For example, if you want to install the
tidyverse package then click the Install button. Please make sure that you need to
have internet access to do this. You can also install packages from:

- a zip file (from your machine or USB)
- from github repository
- other repository

2.5   Working Directory

Setting and knowing the R working directory is very important. Our working directory will contain the R codes, the R outputs, datasets or even resources or tutorials that can help us during in R project or during our R analysis/

The working directory is just a folder. Moreover, the folder can contain many subfolders. We recommend that the folder contain the dataset (if you want to analyze your data locally) and other R objects. R will store many other R objects created during each R session.

Type this to locate the working directory:

```
getwd()
```

```
## [1] "C:/Users/drkim/Downloads/multivar_data_analysis/multivar_data_analysis"
```

2.5.1   Starting a new R job

There are two ways to start a new R job:

- create a new R project from RStudio IDE. This is the method that we recommend.
- setting your working directory using the `setwd()` function.

2.5.2   Creating a new R project

We highly encourage users to create a new R project. To do this, users can

- go to `File -> New Project`

When you see project type, click New Project

2.5.3   Location for dataset

Many data analysts use data stored on their local machines. R will read data and usually store this data in data frame format or class. When you read your data into RStudio, you will see the dataset in the environment pane. RStudio reads the original dataset and saves it to the RAM (random access memory). So you must know the size of your computer RAM. How much is your RAM for your machine? The bigger the RAM, the larger R can read and store your data in the computer's memory.

The data read (in memory) will disappear once you close RStudio. But the source dataset will stay in its original location, so there will be no change to your original data (be happy!) unless you save the data frame in the memory and replace the original file. However, we do not recommend you do this.

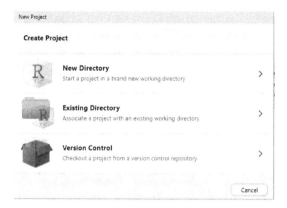

FIGURE 2.6
New Project.

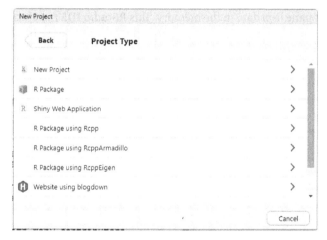

FIGURE 2.7
Project type.

2.6 Upload Data to RStudio Cloud

If users want to use data in the RStuio Cloud, they may have to upload the data to the RStudio Cloud directory. They may also use RStudio Cloud to read data from the **Dropbox** folder or **Google Drive** folder.

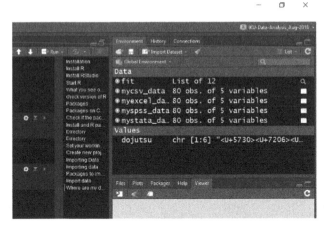

FIGURE 2.8
Environment pane lists data in the memory. This RStudio IDE interface uses the Vibrant Ink theme which users can choose from the Appearance tab in Global Option menu inside the Tools tab.

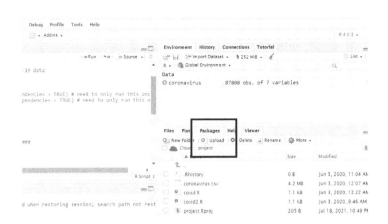

FIGURE 2.9
Upload tab on RStudio Cloud.

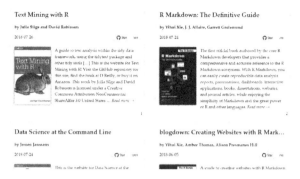

FIGURE 2.10
Examples of two books that are freely accessible on the Bookdown website and also available as physical books.

2.7 More Resources on RStudio Cloud

There are a number of resources on RStudio Cloud. For example, on YouTube channel, there is RStudio Cloud for Education https://www.youtube.com/watch?v =PviVimazpz8. Another good resource on YouTube is Working with R in Cloud https://www.youtube.com/watch?v=SFpzr21Pavg

2.8 Guidance and Help

To see further guidance and help, users may register and join RStudio Community at RStudio Community[3]. Users can also ask questions on Stack Overflow[4]. There are also mailing list groups on specific topics but users have to subscribe to it.

2.9 Bookdown

RStudio has provided a website to host online books, the Bookdown[5]. The books at Bookdown are freely accessible online. There are some of the books that are available on Amazon or other book depository as physical books such as ours.

---

[3] https://community.rstudio.com/
[4] https://stackoverflow.com/
[5] https://bookdown.org/

2.10   Summary

In this chapter, we describe R scripts and R packages. We also show how to write simple R scripts and how to check if any specific R package is available on your machine and how to install it if it is not available. We recommend using RStudio Cloud if you are very new to R. Working directory sometimes confuses new R users, hence we also recommend all R users to create new RStudio Project for new analysis task. There are resources available offline and online and many of them are freely accessible especially at the Bookdown[6] website.

---

[6]https://bookdown.org/

3

RStudio Project

3.1 Objectives

At the end of the chapter, we expect readers to be able to:

- link their RStudio with our datasets. The datasets are on our GitHub repository
- create an RStudio Cloud project using our GitHub repository
- create an RStudio project on a local machine using our GitHub repository

---

3.2 Introduction

In this chapter, we will guide you to have a similar folder and file structure to our project for this book. This folder and file structure will help you run the codes with minimal error risk. Furthermore, to achieve this, we will use the RStudio Project.

On the RStudio Project webpage[1], it says that RStudio projects make it straightforward to divide your work into multiple contexts, each with their working directory, workspace, history and source documents.RStudio projects are associated with R working directories. You can create an RStudio project:

- on RStudio Cloud or RStudio on your local machine
- In a brand new directory
- In an existing directory where you already have R code and data
- By cloning a version control (Git or Subversion) repository

---

[1]https://support.rstudio.com/hc/en-us/articles/200526207-Using-RStudio-Projects

DOI: 10.1201/9781003296775-3

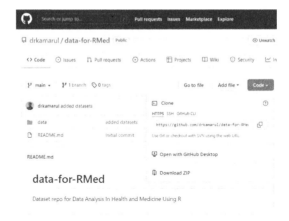

FIGURE 3.1
The dataset repository on GitHub.

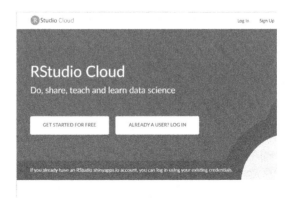

FIGURE 3.2
RStudio Cloud.

3.3 Dataset Repository on GitHub

We will use the our GitHub repository that contains the book's datasets. The name of the repository is data-for-RMed. To go to the repository, click on this link[2]

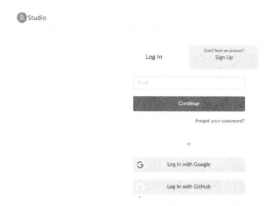

FIGURE 3.3
RStudio Cloud login page.

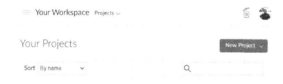

FIGURE 3.4
Rstudio Cloud, Workspace and New Project.

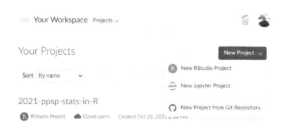

FIGURE 3.5
New Project from the Git repository.

3.4 RStudio Project on RStudio or Posit Cloud

Rstudio Cloud is now known as Posit Cloud. With RStudio and Posit Cloud, you can easily and conveniently access RStudio IDE. In this section, we will show you how to create a RStudio or Posit Cloud project copied from our book repository on the GitHub. We advise you to follow these steps:

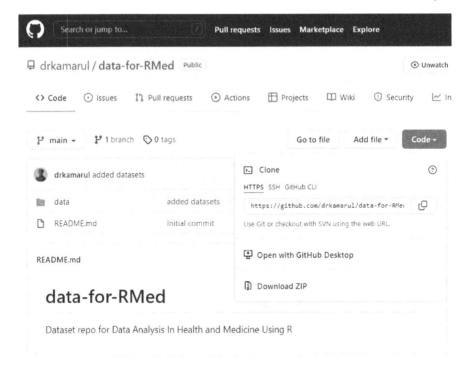

FIGURE 3.6
Clone the dataset repository to RStudio Cloud.

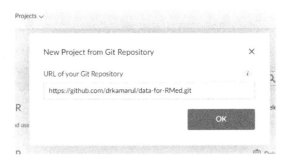

FIGURE 3.7
Cloning the GitHub repository on RStudio or Posit Cloud project by pasting the HTTPS GitHub repository link.

- Go to your RStudio Cloud login page.
- Next, log in to your RStudio or Posit Cloud using your credentials.
- Once inside your work space, click **New Project**.
- Click on the **New Project from Git Repository**.

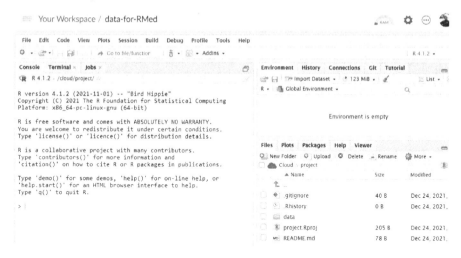

FIGURE 3.8
A new RStudio Cloud Project.

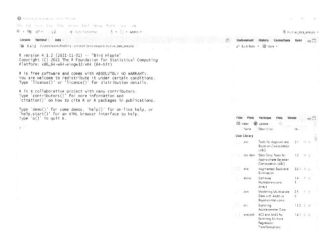

FIGURE 3.9
RStudio on Your Machine.

- After you have clicked the New Project, go back to our **data-for-RMed** repository on GitHub.

- Click on **Clone** button.

- Then click the copy button for **HTTPS**.

- Paste the copied HTTPS link. You have just cloned the repository to your RStudio or Posit Cloud. This will ensure your file structure is the same as that of our RStudio or Posit Cloud.

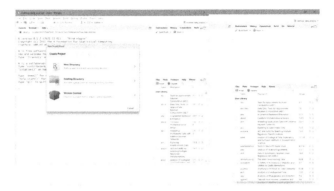

FIGURE 3.10
New Project Wizard.

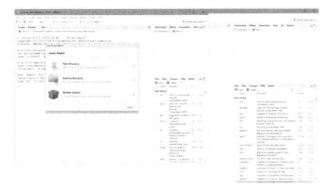

FIGURE 3.11
New Project Wizard and Version Control.

- Then, click OK.

What you will see on your screen is a new Rstudio Cloud project. It will read **Your Workspace**, and the directory name is **data-for-RMed**

3.5   RStudio Project on Local Machine

The steps are rather similar if you want to create a new project on your local machine using the same GitHub repository.

Below, we list the steps that you can follow to create a new project based on our GitHub repository:

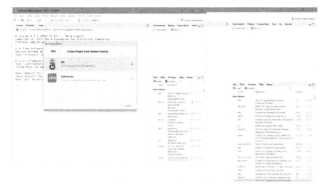

FIGURE 3.12
Git on the Create Project from Version Control tab.

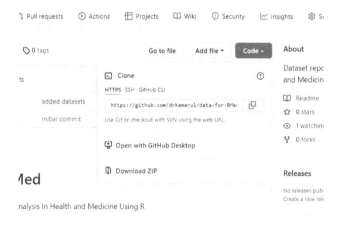

FIGURE 3.13
Copy the HTTPS from GitHub.

- Start your RStudio IDE.

- On the menu, click **File**, then click **New Project**.

- Next, click **Project** and then click **Version Control**.

- After that, you click **Git**.

- As you remember from the previous step where we copied GitHub HTTPS link. So it is the same step here; Copy the HTTPS link from **dataset-for-RMed** GitHub repository.

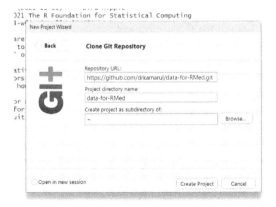

FIGURE 3.14
Clone Git Repository.

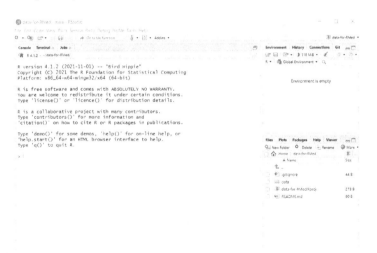

FIGURE 3.15
A new RStudio project.

- Now, you can paste the HTTPS link (see Figure 3.14). You will notice that the **Project directory name** will be automatically filled. You can next click on **Browse**, so that you can choose whichever folder that you prefer to be your working directory.

We recommend you using your home directory (such as **Documents** if you are using Microsoft Windows OS).

And now you will notice that RStudio will create a new working directory on your local machine. This working directory contains the same folder and file structures with the our GitHub repository:

3.6 Summary

In this chapter, we showed to readers how to set their R environment so they will the produce same folder and file structures in their RStudio working directory similar to ours. By using this strategy, we will minimize the errors the readers are making when they are the R codes from our book. We also show the location of the datasets. They are originally stored on the GitHub repository for this book. Then, we provided the instructions to readers so they are able to create new RStudio projects on Posit Cloud (previously known as RStudio Cloud) remotely and on their RStudio IDE on the local machines.

4

Data Visualization

4.1 Objectives

In this chapter, readers will:

- be introduced to the concept of data visualization
- be able to understand the ingredients for good graphics
- be able to generate plots using **ggplot** packages
- be able to save plots in different formats and graphical settings

In our physical book, the plots will be published in black and white text. Because of that, some of the R codes that come with **ggplot2** will have an additional line of codes such as `scale_colour_grey() +` and `scale_line_grey()` to make sure the plots suit the black and white text inside our physical book. The online version of our book on the bookdown website[1] shows the plots in color.

4.2 Introduction

Many disciplines view data visualization as a modern equivalent of visual communication. It involves the creation and study of the visual representation of data. Data visualization requires "information that has been abstracted in some schematic form, including attributes or variables for the units of information". You can read more about data visualization on this wikipedia[2] page and another wikipedia[3] page.

---

[1]https://bookdown.org/drki_musa/dataanalysis/
[2]https://en.m.wikipedia.org/wiki/Data_visualization
[3]https://en.m.wikipedia.org/wiki/Michael_Friendly

DOI: 10.1201/9781003296775-4

4.3   History and Objectives of Data Visualization

In his 1983 book, which carried the title *The Visual Display of Quantitative Informa-tion*, the author Edward Tufte defines **graphical displays** and principles for effective graphical display. The book mentioned, "Excellence in statistical graphics consists of complex ideas communicated with clarity, precision and efficiency".

Visualization is the process of representing data graphically and interacting with these representations. The objective is to gain insight into the data. Some of the pro-cesses are outlined on Watson IBM webpage[4]

4.4   Ingredients for Good Graphics

Good graphics are essential to convey the message from your data visually. They will complement the text for your books, reports or manuscripts. However, you need to make sure that while writing codes for graphics, you need to consider these ingredi-ents:

- You have good data
- Priorities on substance rather than methodology, graphic design, the technology of graphic production or something else
- Do not distort what the data has to say
- Show the presence of many numbers in a small space
- Coherence for large data sets
- Encourage the eye to compare different pieces of data
- Graphics reveal data at several levels of detail, from a broad overview to the fine structure
- Graphics serve a reasonably clear purpose: description, exploration, tabulation or decoration
- Be closely integrated with a data set's statistical and verbal descriptions.

4.5   Graphics Packages in R

There are several packages to create graphics in R. They include packages that per-form general data visualization or graphical tasks. The others provide specific graph-ics for certain statistical or data analyses.

---

[4]http://researcher.watson.ibm.com/researcher/view_group.php?id=143

The popular general-purpose graphics packages in R include:

- **graphics** : a base R package, which means it is loaded every time we open R
- **ggplot2** : a user-contributed package by RStudio, so you must install it the first time you use it. It is a standalone package but also comes together with **tidyverse** package
- **lattice** : This is a user-contributed package. It provides the ability to display multivariate relationships, and it improves on the base-R graphics. This package supports the creation of trellis graphs: graphs that display a variable or.

A few examples of more specific graphical packages include:

- **survminer** : The **survminer** R package provides functions for facilitating survival analysis and visualization. It contains the function `ggsurvplot()` for drawing easily beautiful and ready-to-publish survival curves with the *number at risk* table and *censoring count plot*.
- **sjPlot** : Collection of plotting and table output functions for data visualization. Using **sjPlot**, you can make plots for various statistical analyses including simple and cross-tabulated frequencies, histograms, box plots, (generalized) linear models, mixed effects models, principal component analysis and correlation matrices, cluster analyses, scatter plots, stacked scales, and effects plots of regression models (including interaction terms).

Except for **graphics** package (a base R package), other packages such as **ggplot2** and **lattice** need to be installed into your R library if you want to use them for the first time.

4.6   The ggplot2 Package

We will focus on using the **ggplot2** package for this book. The **ggplot2** package is an elegant, easy and versatile general graphics package in R. It implements the **grammar of graphics** concept. This concept's advantage is that it fastens the process of learning graphics. It also facilitates the process of creating complex graphics

To work with **ggplot2**, remember that at least your R codes must

- start with `ggplot()`
- identify which data to plot `data = Your Data`
- state variables to plot for example `aes(x = Variable on x-axis, y = Variable on y-axis )` for bivariate
- choose type of graph, for example `geom_histogram()` for histogram, and `geom_points()` for scatterplots

The official website for ggplot2 is here https://ggplot2.tidyverse.org/ which is an excellent resource. The website states that *ggplot2* is a plotting system for R, based on the grammar of graphics, which tries to take the good parts of base and lattice graphics and none of the bad parts. It takes care of many fiddly details that make plotting a hassle (like drawing legends) and provides a powerful model of graphics that makes it easy to produce complex multi-layered graphics.

4.7 Preparation

4.7.1 Create a new RStudio project

We always recommend that whenever users want to start working on a new data analysis project in RStudio, they should create a new R project.

- Go to `File,`
- Click `New Project.`

If you want to create a new R project using an existing folder, then choose this folder directory when requested in the `existing Directory` in the `New Project Wizard` window. An R project directory is useful because RStudio will store and save your codes and outputs in that directory (folder).

If you do not want to create a new project, then ensure you are inside the correct directory (R call this a working directory). The working directory is a folder where you store your codes and outputs. If you want to locate your working directory, type `getwd()` in your Console.

Inside your working directory,

- we recommend you keep your dataset and your codes (R scripts `.R`, R markdown files `.Rmd`)
- RStudio will store your outputs

4.7.2 Important questions before plotting graphs

It would be best if you asked yourselves these:

- Which variable or variables do you want to plot?
- What is (or are) the type of that variable?
  - Are they factor (categorical) variables or numerical variables?
- Am I going to plot
  - a single variable?
  - two variables together?
  - three variables together?

4.8   Read Data

R can read almost all (if not all) types of data. The common data formats in data and statistical analysis include

- comma-separated files (.csv)
- MS Excel file (.xlsx)
- SPSS file (.sav)
- Stata file (.dta)
- SAS file (.sas)

However, it would help if you had user-contributed packages to read data from statistical software. For example. **haven** and **rio** packages.

Below we show the functions to read SAS, SPSS and Stata files using the **haven** package.

1. SAS: read_sas() reads .sas7bdat + .sas7bcat files and read_xpt() reads SAS transport files (version 5 and version 8). write_sas() writes .sas7bdat files.
2. SPSS: read_sav() reads .sav files and read_por() reads the older .por files. write_sav() writes .sav files.
3. Stata: read_dta() reads .dta files (up to version 15). write_dta() writes .dta files (versions 8-15).

Sometimes, users may want to analyze data stored in databases. Some examples of common databases format are:

1. MySQL
2. SQLite
3. Postgresql
4. MariaDB

To read data from databases, you must connect your RStudio IDE with the database. There is an excellent resource to do this on the *Databases Using R* webpage[5]

4.9   Load the Packages

The **ggplot2** package is one of the core member of **tidyverse** metapackage (https://www.tidyverse.org/). So, whenever we load the **tidyverse** package, we automatically

---

[5]https://solutions.rstudio.com/db/

load other packages inside the **tidyverse** metapackage. These packages include **dplyr**, **readr** and of course **ggplot2**.

Loading a package will give you access to

1. help pages of the package
2. functions available in the package
3. sample datasets (not all packages contain this feature)

We also load the **here** package in the example below. This package is helpful to point R codes to the specific folder of an R project directory. We will see this in action later.

```
library(tidyverse)
```

```
## -- Attaching core tidyverse packages ----------------------- tidyverse 2.0.0 -
-
## v dplyr      1.1.1      v readr      2.1.4
## v forcats    1.0.0      v stringr    1.5.0
## v ggplot2    3.4.2      v tibble     3.2.1
## v lubridate  1.9.2      v tidyr      1.3.0
## v purrr      1.0.1
##          --        Conflicts      ----------------------------------------
tidyverse_conflicts() --
## x dplyr::filter() masks stats::filter()
## x dplyr::lag()    masks stats::lag()
##      i     Use     the     conflicted     package     (<http://conflicted.r-
lib.org/>) to force all conflicts to become errors
```

```
library(here)
```

```
## here() starts at C:/Users/drkim/Downloads/multivar_data_analysis/multivar_data_analysis
```

If you run the library() code and then get this message *there is no package called tidyverse*, it means the package is still unavailable in your R library. So, you need to install the missing package. Similarly, if you receive the error message while loading the **tidyverse** package, you must install it.

To install an R package for example **tidyverse**, type install.package("tidyverse") in the Console. Once the installation is complete, type library(tidyverse) again to load the package. Alternatively, you can use the GUI to install the package.

Now, type the package you want to install. For example, if you want to install the **tidyverse** package, then type the name in the box.

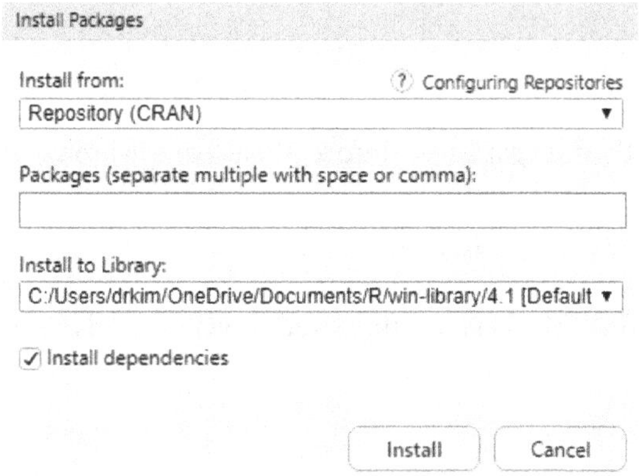

FIGURE 4.1
Packages window.

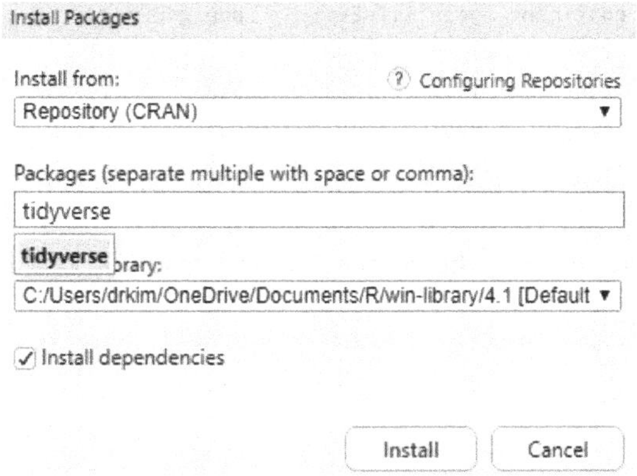

FIGURE 4.2
Typing name of the package to install.

4.10 Read the Dataset

In this chapter, we will use two datasets, the gapminder dataset and a peptic ulcer dataset. The gapminder dataset is a built-in dataset in the **gapminder** package. You can read more about *gapminder* from https://www.gapminder.org/ webpage. The gapminder website contains many useful datasets and shows excellent graphics, made popular by the late Dr Hans Rosling.

To load the **gapminder** package, type:

```
library(gapminder)
```

Next, we will call the data *gapminder* into R. Then , we will browse the first six observations of the data. The codes below:

- assigns gapminder as a dataset
- contains a pipe %>% that connects two codes (gapminder and slice)
- contains a function called slice() that selects rows of the dataset

```
gapminder <- gapminder
gapminder %>%
  slice(1:4)
```

```
## # A tibble: 4 x 6
##    country     continent  year lifeExp      pop gdpPercap
##    <fct>       <fct>     <int>   <dbl>    <int>     <dbl>
## 1 Afghanistan Asia       1952    28.8  8425333      779.
## 2 Afghanistan Asia       1957    30.3  9240934      821.
## 3 Afghanistan Asia       1962    32.0 10267083      853.
## 4 Afghanistan Asia       1967    34.0 11537966      836.
```

It is a good idea to quickly list the variables of the dataset and look at the type of each of the variables:

```
glimpse(gapminder)
```

```
## Rows: 1,704
## Columns: 6
## $ country   <fct> "Afghanistan", "Afghanistan", "Afghanistan", "Afghanistan", ~
## $ continent <fct> Asia, Asia, Asia, Asia, Asia, Asia, Asia, Asia, Asia, Asia, ~
## $ year      <int> 1952, 1957, 1962, 1967, 1972, 1977, 1982, 1987, 1992, 1997, ~
## $ lifeExp   <dbl> 28.801, 30.332, 31.997, 34.020, 36.088, 38.438, 39.854, 40.8~
## $ pop       <int> 8425333, 9240934, 10267083, 11537966, 13079460, 14880372, 12~
## $ gdpPercap <dbl> 779.4453, 820.8530, 853.1007, 836.1971, 739.9811, 786.1134, ~
```

We can see that the *gapminder* dataset has:

- six (6) variables
- a total of 1704 observations
- two factor variables, two integer variables and two numeric (dbl) variables

We can generate some basic statistics of the gapminder datasets by using summary(). This function will list

- the frequencies

- central tendencies and dispersion such as min, first quartile, median, mean, third
  quartile and max

```
summary(gapminder)
```

```
##          country          continent        year          lifeExp
## Afghanistan:  12    Africa   :624   Min.   :1952   Min.   :23.60
## Albania    :  12    Americas:300   1st Qu.:1966   1st Qu.:48.20
## Algeria    :  12    Asia     :396   Median :1980   Median :60.71
## Angola     :  12    Europe   :360   Mean   :1980   Mean   :59.47
## Argentina  :  12    Oceania  : 24   3rd Qu.:1993   3rd Qu.:70.85
## Australia  :  12                    Max.   :2007   Max.   :82.60
## (Other)    :1632
##       pop              gdpPercap
## Min.   :6.001e+04   Min.    :   241.2
## 1st Qu.:2.794e+06   1st Qu.:  1202.1
## Median :7.024e+06   Median :   3531.8
## Mean   :2.960e+07   Mean    :  7215.3
## 3rd Qu.:1.959e+07   3rd Qu.:  9325.5
## Max.   :1.319e+09   Max.    :113523.1
##
```

4.11   Basic Plots

Let us start by creating a simple plot using these arguments:

- data : data = gapminder
- variables : x = year, y = lifeExp
- graph scatterplot : geom_point()

ggplot2 uses the + sign to connect between functions, including **ggplot2** functions
that span multiple lines.

```
ggplot(data = gapminder) +
  geom_point(mapping = aes(x = year, y = lifeExp)) +
  theme_bw()
```

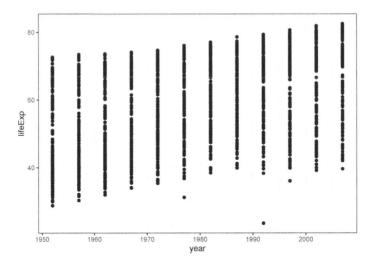

From the plot, we can see

- a scatterplot
- the scatterplot shows the relationship between year and life expectancy
- as variable year advances, the life expectancy increases

If you look closely, you will notice that

- ggplot() function tells R to be ready to make a plot from specified data
- geom_point() function tells R to make a scatter plot

Users may find more resources about **ggplot2** package on the **ggplot2** webpage[6] (Wickham et al., 2020). Other excellent resources include the online R Graphics Cookbook[7] and its physical book (Chang, 2013) .

4.12   More Complex Plots

4.12.1   Adding another variable

We can see that the variables we want to plot are specified by aes(). We can add a third variable to make a more complex plot. For example:

- data : data = gapminder
- variables : x = year, y = lifeExp, colour = continent

---

[6]https://ggplot2.tidyverse.org/reference/ggplot.html
[7]https://r-graphics.org/

The objective of creating plot using multiple (more than two variables) is to enable users to visualize a more complex relationship between more than two variables. Let us take a visualization for variable year, variable life expectancy and variable continent.

This book uses black and white text, so we add the scale_colour_grey() + codes. If readers want to see the color of the plot, just delete this line scale_colour_grey() +.

```
ggplot(data = gapminder) +
  geom_point(mapping = aes(x = year,
                           y = lifeExp,
                           colour = continent)) +
  scale_colour_grey() +
  theme_bw()
```

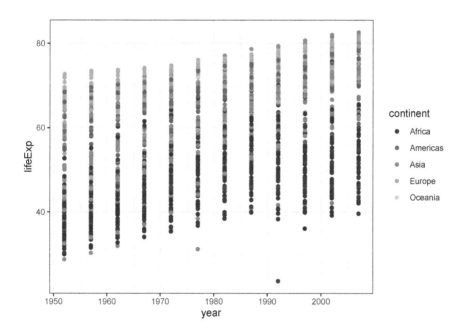

From the scatterplot of these three variables, you may notice that.

- European countries have a high life expectancy
- African countries have a lower life expectancy
- One country is Asia looks like an outlier (very low life expectancy)
- One country in Africa looks like an outlier too (very low life expectancy)

Now, we will replace the third variable with Gross Domestic Product gdpPercap and correlates it with the size of gdpPerCap.

```
ggplot(data = gapminder) +
  geom_point(mapping = aes(x = year,
                           y = lifeExp,
                           size = gdpPercap)) +
  theme_bw()
```

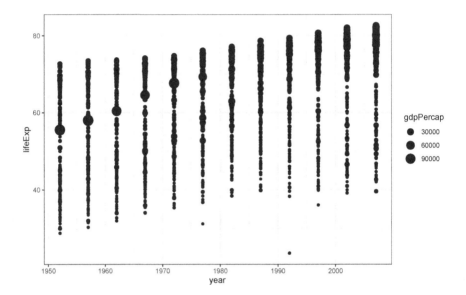

You will notice that *ggplot2* automatically assigns a unique level of the aesthetic (here, a unique color) to each value of the variable, a process known as scaling. *ggplot2* also adds a legend that explains which levels correspond to which values. For example, the plot suggests that with higher gdpPerCap, there is also a longer lifeExp.

Instead of using color, we can also use different shapes. Different shapes are helpful, especially when there is no facility to print out colorful plots. And we use geom_jitter() to disperse the points away from one another. The argument alpha= will set the opacity of the points. However, readers still have difficulty to notice the difference between continents.

```
ggplot(data = gapminder) +
  geom_jitter(mapping = aes(x = year,
                            y = lifeExp,
                            shape = continent),
              width = 0.75, alpha = 0.5) +
  theme_bw()
```

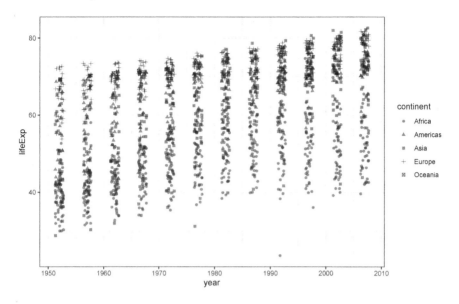

To change the parameter shape, for example, to the plus symbol, you can set the argument for shape to equal 3.

```
ggplot(data = gapminder) +
  geom_point(mapping = aes(x = year, y = lifeExp),
             shape = 3) +
  theme_bw()
```

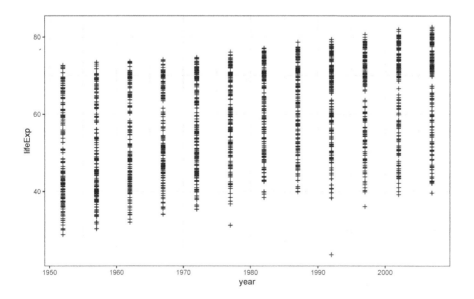

You may be interested to know what number corresponds to what type of shape. To do so, you can type ?pch to access the help document. You will see in the Viewer pane, there will be a document that explains various shapes available in R. It also shows what number that represents each shape.

4.12.2　Making subplots

You can split our plots based on a factor variable and make subplots using the facet(). For example, if we want to make subplots based on continents, then we need to set these parameters:

- data = gapminder
- variable year on the x-axis and lifeExp on the y-axis
- split the plot based on continent
- set the number of rows for the plot at 3

```
ggplot(data = gapminder) +
  geom_point(mapping = aes(x = year, y = lifeExp)) +
  facet_wrap(~ continent, nrow = 3) +
  theme_bw()
```

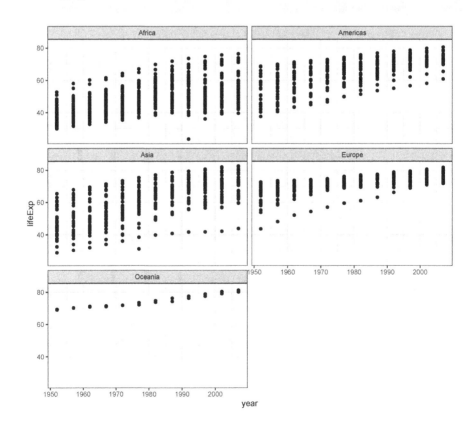

However, you will get a different arrangement of plot, if you change the value for the
nrow

```
ggplot(data = gapminder) +
  geom_point(mapping = aes(x = year, y = lifeExp)) +
  facet_wrap(~ continent, nrow = 2) +
  theme_bw()
```

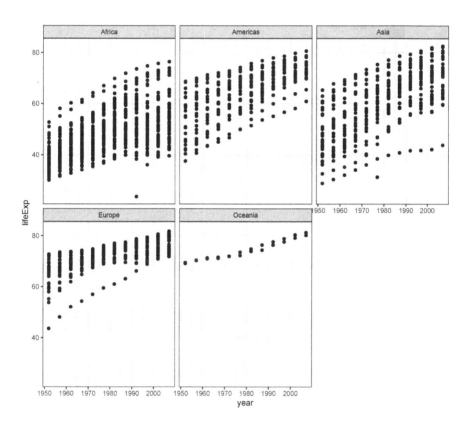

4.12.3 Overlaying plots

Each geom_X() in ggplot2 indicates different visual objects. This is a scatterplot and
we set in R code chuck the fig.width= equals 6 and fig.height= equals 5 (*fig.width=6, fig.height=5*)

```
ggplot(data = gapminder) +
  geom_point(mapping = aes(x = gdpPercap, y = lifeExp)) +
  theme_bw()
```

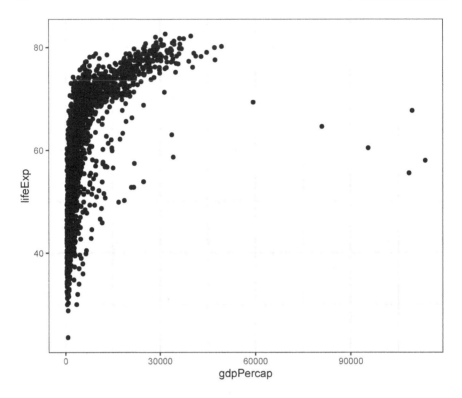

This is a smooth line plot:

```
ggplot(data = gapminder) +
  geom_smooth(mapping = aes(x = gdpPercap, y = lifeExp)) +
  theme_bw()
```

```
## `geom_smooth()` using method = 'gam' and formula = 'y ~ s(x, bs = "cs")'
```

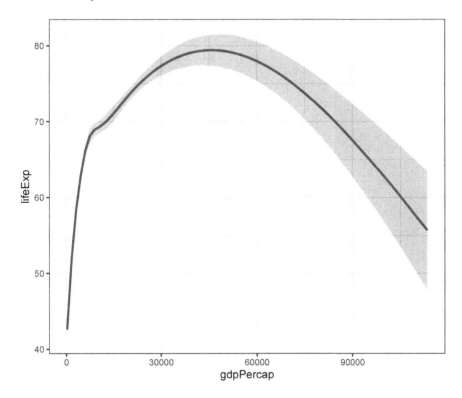

Let's generate a smooth plot based on continent using the `linetype()` and use `log(gdpPercap)` to reduce the skewness of the data. Use these codes:

```
ggplot(data = gapminder) +
  geom_smooth(mapping = aes(x = log(gdpPercap),
                            y = lifeExp,
                            linetype = continent)) +
  theme_bw()
```

```
## `geom_smooth()` using method = 'loess' and formula = 'y ~ x'
```

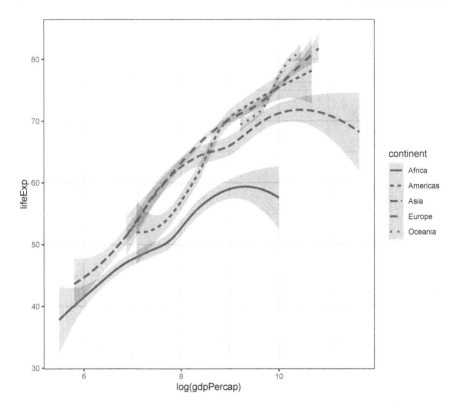

Another smooth plot but setting the parameter for color but in greyscale. Again, if you print on black and white text, and you will not be able to see the color. To see the color clearly, just remove the `scale_colour_grey()` + codes.

```
ggplot(data = gapminder) +
  geom_smooth(mapping = aes(x = log(gdpPercap),
                            y = lifeExp,
                            colour = continent)) +
  scale_colour_grey() +
  theme_bw()
```

```
## `geom_smooth()` using method = 'loess' and formula = 'y ~ x'
```

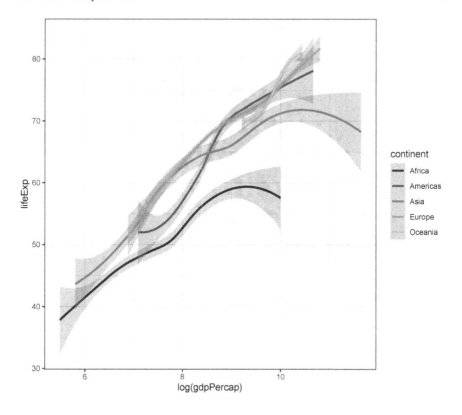

4.12.4   Combining different plots

We can combine more than one geoms (type of plots) to overlay plots. The trick is to use multiple geoms in a single line of R code:

```
ggplot(data = gapminder) +
  geom_point(mapping = aes(x = log(gdpPercap), y = lifeExp)) +
  geom_smooth(mapping = aes(x = log(gdpPercap), y = lifeExp)) +
  theme_bw()


## `geom_smooth()` using method = 'gam' and formula = 'y ~ s(x, bs = "cs")'
```

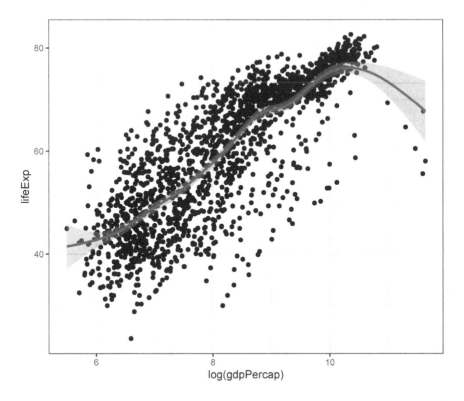

The codes above show duplication or repetition. To avoid this, we can pass the mapping to ggplot():

```
ggplot(data = gapminder,
        mapping = aes(x = log(gdpPercap), y = lifeExp)) +
  geom_point() +
  geom_smooth() +
  theme_bw()
```

```
## `geom_smooth()` using method = 'gam' and formula = 'y ~ s(x, bs = "cs")'
```

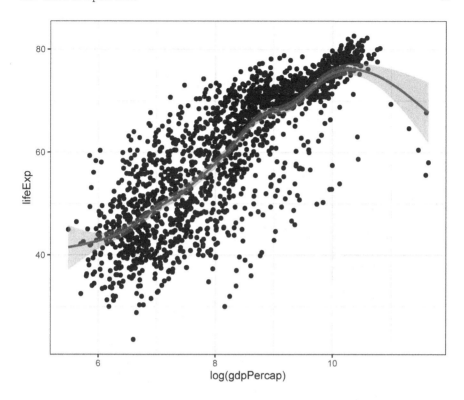

And we can expand this to make scatterplot showing different shapes for the continent:

```
ggplot(data = gapminder,
       mapping = aes(x = log(gdpPercap), y = lifeExp)) +
  geom_point(mapping = aes(shape = continent)) +
  geom_smooth() +
  theme_bw()
```

```
## `geom_smooth()` using method = 'gam' and formula = 'y ~ s(x, bs = "cs")'
```

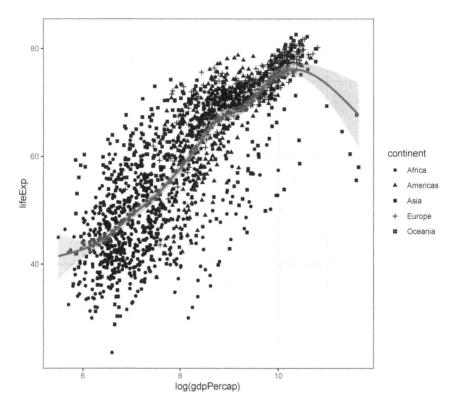

Or expand this to make the smooth plot shows different linetypes for the continent:

```
ggplot(data = gapminder,
       mapping = aes(x = log(gdpPercap), y = lifeExp)) +
  geom_point() +
  geom_smooth(mapping = aes(linetype = continent)) +
  theme_bw()
```

```
## `geom_smooth()` using method = 'loess' and formula = 'y ~ x'
```

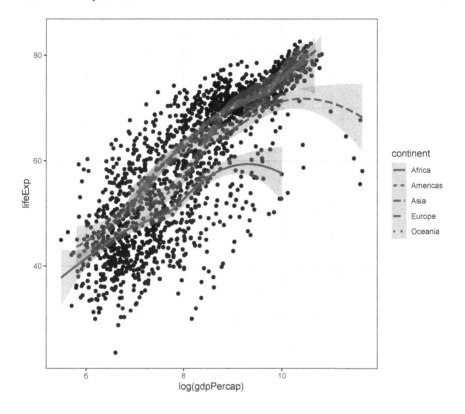

Or both the scatterplot and the smoothplot:

```
ggplot(data = gapminder,
       mapping = aes(x = log(gdpPercap), y = lifeExp)) +
  geom_point(mapping = aes(shape = continent)) +
  geom_smooth(mapping = aes(colour = continent)) +
  scale_colour_grey() +
  theme_bw()
```

```
## `geom_smooth()` using method = 'loess' and formula = 'y ~ x'
```

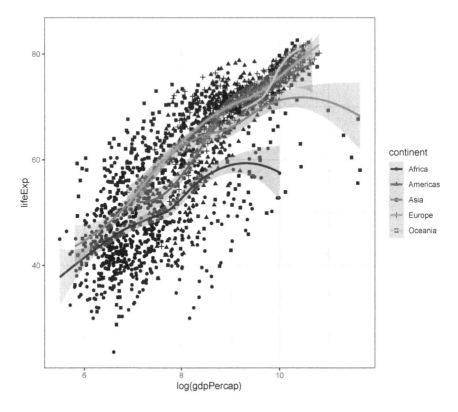

4.12.5   Statistical transformation

Let us create a Bar chart, with y-axis as the frequency.

```
ggplot(data = gapminder) +
  geom_bar(mapping = aes(x = continent)) +
  scale_colour_grey() +
  theme_bw()
```

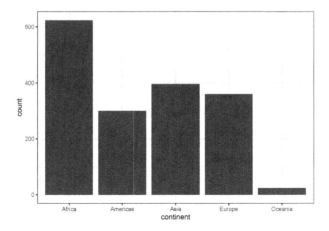

If we want the y-axis to show proportion, we can use these codes.

```
ggplot(data = gapminder) +
  geom_bar(mapping = aes(x = continent, y = after_stat(count/sum(count)),
                    group = 1))
```

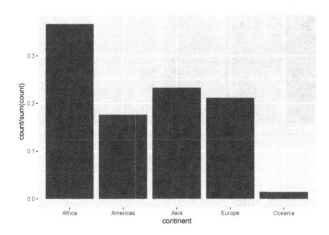

Or you can be more elaborate like below:

```
gapminder2 <-
  gapminder %>%
  count(continent) %>%
  mutate(perc = n/sum(n) * 100)
```

```
pl <- gapminder2 %>%
  ggplot(aes(x = continent, y = n, fill = continent))
pl <- pl + geom_col() + scale_fill_grey(start = 0, end = .9)
pl <- pl + geom_text(aes(x = continent, y = n,
                         label = paste0(n, " (", round(perc,1),"%)"),
                         vjust = -0.5))
pl <- pl + theme_classic()
pl <- pl + labs(title ="Bar chart showing counts and percentages")
pl
```

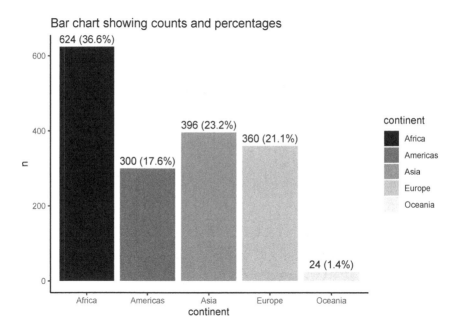

4.12.6   Customizing title

We can customize many aspects of the plot using **ggplot2** package. For example, from gapminder dataset, we choose gdpPerCap and log it (to reduce skewness) and lifeExp, and make a scatterplot.

Let's name the plot as mypop

```
mypop <- ggplot(data = gapminder,
                mapping = aes(x = log(gdpPercap),
                              y = lifeExp,
```

```
                                      shape = continent)) +
    geom_point(alpha = 0.4) +
    geom_smooth(mapping = aes(colour = continent), se = FALSE) +
    scale_colour_grey()
mypop
```

```
## `geom_smooth()` using method = 'loess' and formula = 'y ~ x'
```

You will notice that there is no title in the plot, which is not great. To add the title, you can add a function ggtitle():

```
mypop +
    ggtitle("GDP (in log) and life expectancy")
```

```
## `geom_smooth()` using method = 'loess' and formula = 'y ~ x'
```

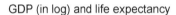

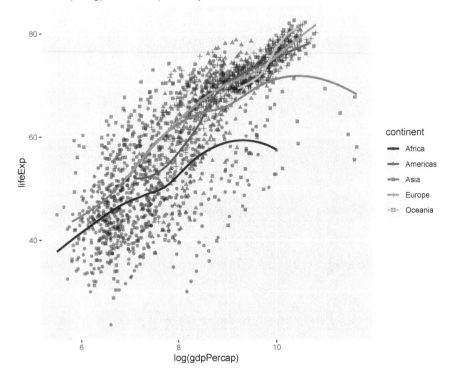

To make the title appears in multiple lines, we can add \n:

```
mypop <- mypop + ggtitle("GDP (in log) and life expectancy:
                \nData from Gapminder")
mypop
```

```
## `geom_smooth()` using method = 'loess' and formula = 'y ~ x'
```

GDP (in log) and life expectancy:

Data from Gapminder

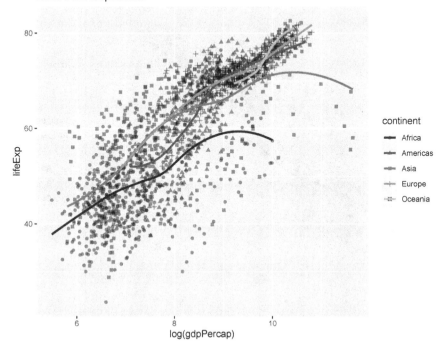

4.12.7 Choosing themes

The default is gray theme or `theme_gray()`. But there are many other themes. One of the popular themes is the black and white theme.

```
mypop <- mypop + theme_bw()
mypop
```

```
## `geom_smooth()` using method = 'loess' and formula = 'y ~ x'
```

GDP (in log) and life expectancy:

Data from Gapminder

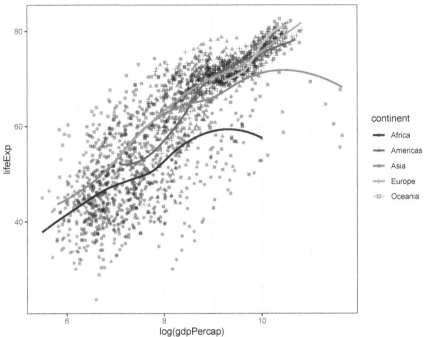

4.12.8   Adjusting axes

We can specify the tick marks, for example:

- min = 0
- max = 12
- interval = 1

```
mypop <- mypop +
  scale_x_continuous(breaks = seq(0,12,1)) +
  scale_y_continuous(breaks = seq(0,90,10))
mypop
```

```
## `geom_smooth()` using method = 'loess' and formula = 'y ~ x'
```

GDP (in log) and life expectancy:

Data from Gapminder

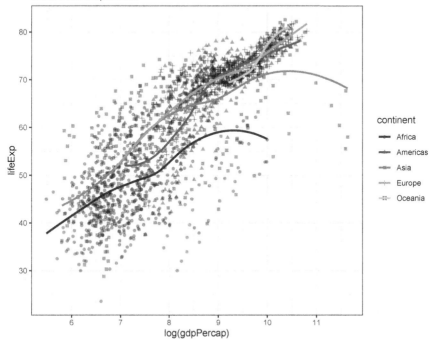

And we can label the x-axis and y-axis:

```
mypop +
  ylab("Life Expentancy") +
  xlab("Percapita GDP in log")
```

```
## `geom_smooth()` using method = 'loess' and formula = 'y ~ x'
```

GDP (in log) and life expectancy:

Data from Gapminder

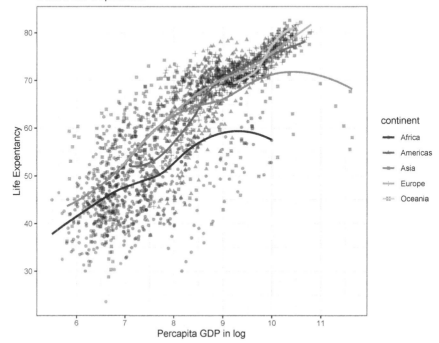

Perhaps, you may want to use `facet_wrap()` to split the plots based on variable continent to show better differences between the plots.

```
ggplot(data = gapminder,
       mapping = aes(x = log(gdpPercap), y = lifeExp)) +
  geom_point(alpha = 0.4) +
  geom_smooth(mapping = aes(line =  continent), se = FALSE) +
  facet_wrap(~ continent) +
  ylab("Life Expentancy") +
  xlab("Percapita GDP in log") +
  theme(legend.position="none") +
  theme_bw()
```

```
## Warning in geom_smooth(mapping = aes(line = continent), se = FALSE): Ignoring
## unknown aesthetics: line
```

```
## `geom_smooth()` using method = 'loess' and formula = 'y ~ x'
```

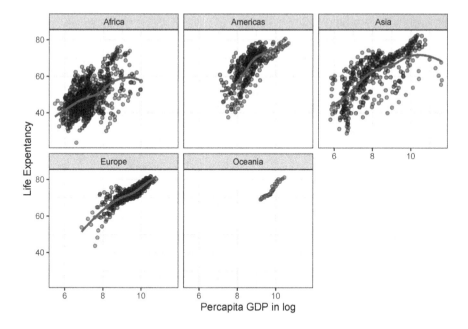

4.13 Saving Plots

In R, you can save the plot in different graphical formats. You can also set other parameters such as the dpi and the size of the plot (height and width). One of the preferred formats for saving a plot is PDF format.

Here, we will show how to save plots in a different format in R. In this example, let us use the object we created before (mypop). We will add

- title
- x label
- y label
- black and white theme

And then create a new graphical object, myplot

```
myplot <-
  mypop +
  ggtitle("GDP (in log) and life expectancy:
             \nData from Gapminder") +
  ylab("Life Expentancy") +
  xlab("Percapita GDP in log") +
```

```
scale_x_continuous(breaks = seq(0,12,1)) +
theme_bw()
```

```
## Scale for x is already present.
## Adding another scale for x, which will replace the existing scale.
```

```
myplot
```

```
## `geom_smooth()` using method = 'loess' and formula = 'y ~ x'
```

GDP (in log) and life expectancy:

Data from Gapminder

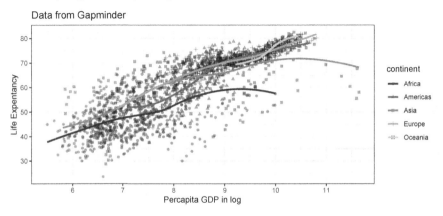

We now can see a nice plot. And next, we want to save the plot (currently on the screen) to these formats:

- pdf format
- png format
- jpg format

If we want to save the plots in a folder named as plots, then

- go to working directory
- click New Folder
- name it as **plot**

This is when the here() function is handy. You can easily point to the correct folder so R knows where to locate the file.

here() is a function under small packages called simply as **here**. This function helps you retrieve or save file or files or r objects from and to the correct path (including folder). This works even when we are using different machines.

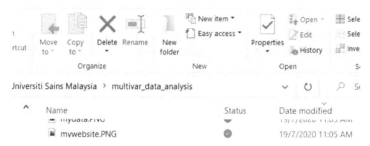

FIGURE 4.3
In Window OS, click the New Folder icon.

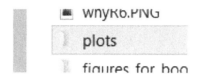

FIGURE 4.4
Rename New Folder as plots.

Many of us recall the uncomfortable experiences when the drive name changes automatically (especially when using a thumb drive) on different computers. By using here() from the **here** package, we will always get to the correct path or folder.

To save the plots in the directory named plots in different image formats, we can do these:

```
ggsave(plot = myplot,
       here("plots","my_pdf_plot.pdf"))


## Saving 6.5 x 4.5 in image
## `geom_smooth()` using method = 'loess' and formula = 'y ~ x'


ggsave(plot = myplot,
       here("plots","my_png_plot.png"))


## Saving 6.5 x 4.5 in image
## `geom_smooth()` using method = 'loess' and formula = 'y ~ x'


ggsave(plot = myplot,
       here("plots","my_jpg_plot.jpg"))
```

```
## Saving 6.5 x 4.5 in image
## `geom_smooth()` using method = 'loess' and formula = 'y ~ x'
```

ggplot2 is flexible and contains many customizations. For example, we want to set these parameters to our plots:

1. width = 10 cm (or you can use in for inches)
2. height = 6 cm (or you can use in for inches)
3. dpi = 150. dpi is dots per inch

```
ggsave(plot = myplot,
       here('plots','my_pdf_plot2.pdf'),
       width = 10, height = 6, units = "in",
       dpi = 150, device = 'pdf')
```

```
## `geom_smooth()` using method = 'loess' and formula = 'y ~ x'
```

```
ggsave(plot = myplot,
       here('plots','my_png_plot2.png'),
       width = 10, height = 6, units = "cm",
       dpi = 150, device = 'png')
```

```
## `geom_smooth()` using method = 'loess' and formula = 'y ~ x'
```

```
ggsave(plot = myplot,
       here("plots","my_jpg_plot2.jpg"),
       width = 10, height = 6, units = "cm",
       dpi = 150, device = 'jpg')
```

```
## `geom_smooth()` using method = 'loess' and formula = 'y ~ x'
```

4.14   Summary

In this chapter, we briefly describe important matters before making plots. Then we teach readers to make plots using the **ggplot2** package. This package uses the principle of Grammar for Graphics to ensure the codes are more intuitive to users. Readers learn to generate a simple plot for one variable before plotting two and three variables simultaneously. **ggplot2** is also flexible and contains many customizations to help readers generate fantastic plots and how to save them.

5

Data Wrangling

5.1 Objectives

At the end of the chapter, readers will be able to

- understand the role of data wrangling
- understand the basic capabilities of **dplyr** package
- acquire skills to perform common data wrangling using **dplyr** and **forcats** packages

5.2 Introduction

Data wrangling removes errors and combines complex data sets to make them more accessible and easier to analyze. Due to the rapid expansion of the amount of data and data sources available today, storing and organizing large quantities of data for analysis is becoming increasingly necessary.

5.2.1 Definition of data wrangling

Data wrangling is also known as Data Munging or Data Transformation. It is loosely the process of manually converting or mapping data from one "raw" form into another format. The process allows for more convenient consumption of the data. You can find more information at mode analytics webpage[1]

Data wrangling sometimes is also referred to as data munging. It is the process of transforming and mapping data from one "raw" data form into another format to make it more appropriate and valuable for various downstream purposes such as analytics. The goal of data wrangling is to ensure quality and valuable data. Data analysts typically spend the majority of their time in the process of data wrangling compared to the actual analysis of the data. Almost all data require data wrangling

---

[1]https://community.modeanalytics.com/sql/tutorial/data-wrangling-with-sql/

DOI: 10.1201/9781003296775-5

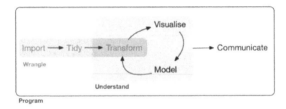

FIGURE 5.1
Main parts of data wrangling.

before further analysis. There are three main parts to data wrangling (Wickham and Grolemund, 2017).

5.3   Data Wrangling with dplyr Package

5.3.1   dplyr package

dplyr is a package grouped inside **tidyverse** collection of packages. **dplyr** package is very useful to munge, wrangle, or transform your data. It is a grammar of data manipulation. It provides a consistent set of verbs that help you solve the most common data manipulation challenges. This **tidyverse** webpage[2] has more information and examples.

5.3.2   Common data wrangling processes

The common data wrangling processes include:

- reducing the size of dataset by selecting certain variables (or columns)
- generating new variable from existing variables
- sorting observation of a variable
- grouping observations based on certain criteria
- reducing variables to groups in order to estimate summary statistic

5.3.3   Some dplyr functions

For the procedures listed above, the corresponding **dplyr** functions are

- `dplyr::select()` – to select a number of variables from a dataframe
- `dplyr::mutate()` – to generate a new variable from existing variables
- `dplyr::arrange()` – to sort observation of a variable
- `dplyr::filter()` – to group observations that fulfill certain criteria

---

[2]https://github.com/tidyverse/dplyr

- `dplyr::group_by()` and `dplyr::summarize()` – to reduce variable to groups in order to provide summary statistic

---

5.4 Preparation

5.4.1 Create a new project or set the working directory

It is essential to ensure you know where your working directory is. The recommended practice *is to create a new project every time you want to start a new analysis with R*. To do so, create a new project by `File -> New Project`. If you do not start with an R new project, you still need to know **the location of your working directory on your computer**.

So, again we emphasize that every time you want to start processing your data, please make sure:

1. use R project. It is much easier and cleaner to start your work with a new R project. Once you have done or need to log off your computer, close the project and reopen the project the next time you need to.

2. if you are not using R project, you are inside the correct working directory. Type `getwd()` to display the active **working directory**. And to set a new working directory, use the function `setwd()`. Once you know where your working directory is, you can start reading or importing data into your working directory.

Once inside the project, you can import your data if necessary.

5.4.2 Load the libraries

Remember, there are several packages you can use to read the data into R. R can read almost all (if not all format) types of data format. For example, we know that common data formats are the:

- SPSS (`.sav`) format,
- Stata (`.dta`) format,
- SAS format,
- MS Excel (`.xlsx`) format
- Comma-separated-values `.csv` format.

However, there are other formats, too, such as data in DICOM format. DICOM format data includes data from CT scans and MRI images. There are data in shapefile format to store geographical information. Three packages - **haven**, **rio**, **readr** and **foreign** packages - are very useful to read or import your data into R memory.

- **readr** provides a fast and friendly way to read rectangular data (like csv, tsv, and fwf). This is contained inside the **tidyverse** metapackage
- **rio** provides a quick way to read almost all type of spreadsheet and statistical software data
- **readxl** reads .xls and .xlsx sheets.
- **haven** reads SPSS, Stata, and SAS data.

We will use the **here** package to facilitate us working with the working directory and **lubridate** to help us wrangle dates.

```
library(tidyverse)
```

```
## -- Attaching core tidyverse packages ---------------------- tidyverse 2.0.0 -
-
## v dplyr     1.1.1      v readr     2.1.4
## v forcats   1.0.0      v stringr   1.5.0
## v ggplot2   3.4.2      v tibble    3.2.1
## v lubridate 1.9.2      v tidyr     1.3.0
## v purrr     1.0.1
##          --         Conflicts          -----------------------------------------
tidyverse_conflicts() --
## x dplyr::filter() masks stats::filter()
## x dplyr::lag()    masks stats::lag()
##     i    Use    the    conflicted    package    (<http://conflicted.r-
lib.org/>) to force all conflicts to become errors
```

```
library(rio)
library(here)
```

```
## here() starts at C:/Users/drkim/Downloads/multivar_data_analysis/multivar_data_analysis
```

```
library(lubridate)
```

When we read datasets with long variable names and spaces - especially after reading the MS Excel dataset - we can use the **janitor** package to generate more R user-friendly variable names.

5.4.3 Datasets

We will use two datasets.

- the stroke dataset in `csv` format
- the peptic ulcer dataset in `xlsx` format

Let's read the datasets and name it, each as

- stroke
- pep

```
stroke <- read_csv(here("data", "stroke_data.csv"))
```

```
## Rows: 213 Columns: 12
## -- Column specification --------------------------------------------
---
## Delimiter: ","
## chr (7): doa, dod, status, sex, dm, stroke_type, referral_from
## dbl (5): gcs, sbp, dbp, wbc, time2
##
## i Use `spec()` to retrieve the full column specification for this data.
## i Specify the column types or set `show_col_types = FALSE` to quiet this message.
```

```
pep <- import(here("data", "peptic_ulcer.xlsx"))
```

Take a peek at the stroke and pep datasets.

The stroke dataset contains:

- 219 observations
- 12 variables

```
glimpse(stroke)
```

```
## Rows: 213
## Columns: 12
## $ doa           <chr> "17/2/2011", "20/3/2011", "9/4/2011", "12/4/2011", "12/4~
## $ dod           <chr> "18/2/2011", "21/3/2011", "10/4/2011", "13/4/2011", "13/~
## $ status        <chr> "alive", "alive", "dead", "dead", "alive", "dead", "aliv~
## $ sex           <chr> "male", "male", "female", "male", "female", "female", "m~
## $ dm            <chr> "no", "no", "no", "no", "yes", "no", "no", "yes", "yes",~
## $ gcs           <dbl> 15, 15, 11, 3, 15, 3, 11, 15, 6, 15, 15, 4, 4, 10, 12, 1~
## $ sbp           <dbl> 151, 196, 126, 170, 103, 91, 171, 106, 170, 123, 144, 23~
## $ dbp           <dbl> 73, 123, 78, 103, 62, 55, 80, 67, 90, 83, 89, 120, 120, ~
## $ wbc           <dbl> 12.5, 8.1, 15.3, 13.9, 14.7, 14.2, 8.7, 5.5, 10.5, 7.2, ~
## $ time2         <dbl> 1, 1, 1, 1, 1, 1, 1, 1, 1, 1, 1, 1, 1, 1, 1, 1, 1, 1, 1,~
## $ stroke_type   <chr> "IS", "IS", "HS", "IS", "IS", "HS", "IS", "IS", "HS", "I~
## $ referral_from <chr> "non-hospital", "non-hospital", "hospital", "hospital", ~
```

The pep datasets contains:

- 121 observations
- 34 variables

```
glimpse(pep)
```

```
## Rows: 121
## Columns: 34
## $ age                 <dbl> 42, 66, 67, 19, 77, 39, 62, 71, 69, 97, 52, 21, 57~
## $ gender              <chr> "male", "female", "male", "male", "male", "male", ~
## $ epigastric_pain     <chr> "yes", "yes", "yes", "yes", "yes", "yes", "yes", "~
## $ vomiting            <chr> "no", "no", "no", "no", "yes", "no", "no", "yes", ~
## $ nausea              <chr> "no", "no", "no", "no", "yes", "no", "no", "no", "~
## $ fever               <chr> "no", "no", "no", "no", "no", "yes", "no", "yes", ~
## $ diarrhea            <chr> "no", "no", "yes", "no", "no", "no", "no", "yes", ~
## $ malena              <chr> "no", "no", "no", "no", "no", "no", "no", "no", "n~
## $ onset_more_24_hrs   <chr> "no", "no", "no", "yes", "yes", "yes", "yes", "no"~
## $ NSAIDS              <chr> "no", "no", "yes", "no", "no", "no", "no", "no", "~
## $ septic_shock        <chr> "no", "no", "no", "no", "no", "no", "no", "no", "n~
## $ previous_OGDS       <chr> "no", "no", "no", "yes", "no", "no", "no", "no", "~
## $ ASA                 <dbl> 1, 1, 1, 1, 2, 1, 2, 2, 1, 1, 2, 1, 2, 1, 1, 2, 2,~
## $ systolic            <dbl> 141, 197, 126, 90, 147, 115, 103, 159, 145, 105, 1~
## $ diastolic           <dbl> 98, 88, 73, 40, 82, 86, 55, 68, 75, 65, 74, 50, 86~
## $ inotropes           <chr> "no", "no", "no", "no", "no", "no", "no", "no", "n~
## $ pulse               <dbl> 109, 126, 64, 112, 89, 96, 100, 57, 86, 100, 109, ~
## $ tenderness          <chr> "generalized", "generalized", "generalized", "loca~
## $ guarding            <chr> "yes", "yes", "yes", "yes", "no", "yes", "yes", "n~
## $ hemoglobin          <dbl> 18.0, 12.0, 12.0, 12.0, 11.0, 18.0, 8.1, 13.3, 11.~
## $ twc                 <dbl> 6.0, 6.0, 13.0, 20.0, 21.0, 4.0, 5.0, 12.0, 6.0, 2~
## $ platelet            <dbl> 415, 292, 201, 432, 324, 260, 461, 210, 293, 592, ~
## $ creatinine          <dbl> 135, 66, 80, 64, 137, 102, 69, 92, 94, 104, 58, 24~
## $ albumin             <chr> "27", "28", "32", "42", "38", "38", "30", "41", "N~
## $ PULP                <dbl> 2, 3, 3, 2, 7, 1, 2, 5, 3, 4, 2, 3, 4, 3, 5, 5, 1,~
## $ admission_to_op_hrs <dbl> 2, 2, 3, 3, 3, 3, 4, 4, 4, 4, 4, 5, 5, 6, 6, 6, 6,~
## $ perforation         <dbl> 0.5, 1.0, 0.5, 0.5, 1.0, 1.0, 3.0, 1.5, 0.5, 1.5, ~
## $ degree_perforation  <chr> "small", "small", "small", "small", "small", "smal~
## $ side_perforation    <chr> "distal stomach", "distal stomach", "distal stomac~
## $ ICU                 <chr> "no", "no", "no", "no", "yes", "no", "yes", "no", ~
## $ SSSI                <chr> "no", "no", "no", "no", "no", "no", "no", "no", "n~
## $ anast_leak          <chr> "no", "no", "no", "no", "no", "no", "no", "no", "n~
## $ sepsis              <chr> "no", "no", "no", "no", "no", "no", "yes", "no", "~
## $ outcome             <chr> "alive", "alive", "alive", "alive", "alive", "aliv~
```

Next, we examine the first five observations of the data. The rest of the observations are not shown. You can also see the types of variables:

- chr (character),
- int (integer),
- dbl (double)

```
stroke %>% slice_head(n = 5)
```

```
## # A tibble: 5 x 12
##   doa       dod       status sex   dm     gcs   sbp   dbp   wbc time2 stroke_type
##   <chr>     <chr>     <chr>  <chr> <chr> <dbl> <dbl> <dbl> <dbl> <dbl> <chr>
## 1 17/2/2011 18/2/2~ alive  male  no       15   151    73  12.5     1 IS
## 2 20/3/2011 21/3/2~ alive  male  no       15   196   123   8.1     1 IS
## 3 9/4/2011  10/4/2~ dead   fema~ no       11   126    78  15.3     1 HS
## 4 12/4/2011 13/4/2~ dead   male  no        3   170   103  13.9     1 IS
## 5 12/4/2011 13/4/2~ alive  fema~ yes      15   103    62  14.7     1 IS
## # i 1 more variable: referral_from <chr>
```

```
pep %>% slice_head(n = 5)
```

```
##   age gender epigastric_pain vomiting nausea fever diarrhea malena
## 1  42   male             yes       no     no    no       no     no
## 2  66 female             yes       no     no    no       no     no
## 3  67   male             yes       no     no    no      yes     no
## 4  19   male             yes       no     no    no       no     no
## 5  77   male             yes      yes    yes    no       no     no
##   onset_more_24_hrs NSAIDS septic_shock previous_OGDS ASA systolic diastolic
## 1                no     no           no            no   1      141        98
## 2                no     no           no            no   1      197        88
## 3                no    yes           no            no   1      126        73
## 4               yes     no           no           yes   1       90        40
## 5               yes     no           no            no   2      147        82
##   inotropes pulse  tenderness guarding hemoglobin twc platelet creatinine
## 1        no   109 generalized      yes         18   6      415        135
## 2        no   126 generalized      yes         12   6      292         66
## 3        no    64 generalized      yes         12  13      201         80
## 4        no   112   localized      yes         12  20      432         64
## 5        no    89 generalized       no         11  21      324        137
##   albumin PULP admission_to_op_hrs perforation degree_perforation
## 1      27    2                   2         0.5              small
## 2      28    3                   2         1.0              small
## 3      32    3                   3         0.5              small
## 4      42    2                   3         0.5              small
## 5      38    7                   3         1.0              small
##   side_perforation    ICU SSSI anast_leak sepsis outcome
## 1   distal stomach     no   no         no     no   alive
```

```
## 2    distal stomach  no    no          no    no    alive
## 3    distal stomach  no    no          no    no    alive
## 4    distal stomach  no    no          no    no    alive
## 5    distal stomach  yes   no          no    no    alive
```

5.5   Select Variables, Generate New Variable and Rename Variable

We will work with these functions.

- `dplyr::select()`
- `dplyr::mutate()` and
- `dplyr::rename()`

5.5.1   Select variables using `dplyr::select()`

When you work with large datasets with many columns, it is sometimes easier to select only the necessary columns to reduce the dataset size. This is possible by creating a smaller dataset (fewer variables). Then you can work on the initial part of data analysis with this smaller dataset. This will greatly help data exploration.

To create smaller datasets, select some of the columns (variables) in the dataset. For example, in `pep` data, we have 34 variables. Let us generate a new dataset named `pep2` with only ten variables ,

```
pep2 <- pep %>%
  dplyr::select(age, systolic, diastolic, perforation, twc,
                          gender, vomiting, malena, ASA, outcome)
glimpse(pep2)
```

```
## Rows: 121
## Columns: 10
## $ age         <dbl> 42, 66, 67, 19, 77, 39, 62, 71, 69, 97, 52, 21, 57, 58, 84~
## $ systolic    <dbl> 141, 197, 126, 90, 147, 115, 103, 159, 145, 105, 113, 92, ~
## $ diastolic   <dbl> 98, 88, 73, 40, 82, 86, 55, 68, 75, 65, 74, 50, 86, 65, 50~
## $ perforation <dbl> 0.5, 1.0, 0.5, 0.5, 1.0, 1.0, 3.0, 1.5, 0.5, 1.5, 1.0, 0.5~
## $ twc         <dbl> 6.0, 6.0, 13.0, 20.0, 21.0, 4.0, 5.0, 12.0, 6.0, 28.0, 11.~
## $ gender      <chr> "male", "female", "male", "male", "male", "male", "female"~
## $ vomiting    <chr> "no", "no", "no", "no", "yes", "no", "no", "yes", "no", "n~
## $ malena      <chr> "no", "no", "no", "no", "no", "no", "no", "no", "no", "no"~
## $ ASA         <dbl> 1, 1, 1, 1, 2, 1, 2, 2, 1, 1, 2, 1, 2, 1, 1, 2, 2, 1, 1, 3~
## $ outcome     <chr> "alive", "alive", "alive", "alive", "alive", "alive", "dea~
```

The new dataset `pep2` is now created. You can see it in the `Environment` pane.

5.5.2 Generate new variable using `mutate()`

With `mutate()`, you can generate a new variable. For example, in the dataset `pep2`, we want to create a new variable named `pulse_pressure` (systolic minus diastolic blood pressure in mmHg).

$$pulse\ pressure = systolic\ BP - diastolic\ BP$$

And let's observe the first five observations:

```
pep2 <- pep2 %>%
  mutate(pulse_pressure = systolic - diastolic)
pep2 %>%
  dplyr::select(systolic, diastolic, pulse_pressure ) %>%
  slice_head(n = 5)
```

```
##    systolic diastolic pulse_pressure
## 1       141        98             43
## 2       197        88            109
## 3       126        73             53
## 4        90        40             50
## 5       147        82             65
```

Now for the stroke dataset, we will convert doa and dod, both character variables, to a variable of the *date* type

```
stroke <- stroke %>%
  mutate(doa = dmy(doa), dod = dmy(dod))
stroke
```

```
## # A tibble: 213 x 12
##    doa        dod        status sex    dm     gcs   sbp   dbp   wbc time2
##    <date>     <date>     <chr>  <chr>  <chr> <dbl> <dbl> <dbl> <dbl> <dbl>
##  1 2011-02-17 2011-02-18 alive  male   no       15   151    73  12.5     1
##  2 2011-03-20 2011-03-21 alive  male   no       15   196   123   8.1     1
##  3 2011-04-09 2011-04-10 dead   female no       11   126    78  15.3     1
##  4 2011-04-12 2011-04-13 dead   male   no        3   170   103  13.9     1
##  5 2011-04-12 2011-04-13 alive  female yes      15   103    62  14.7     1
##  6 2011-05-04 2011-05-05 dead   female no        3    91    55  14.2     1
##  7 2011-05-22 2011-05-23 alive  male   no       11   171    80   8.7     1
##  8 2011-05-23 2011-05-24 alive  female yes      15   106    67   5.5     1
##  9 2011-07-11 2011-07-12 dead   female yes       6   170    90  10.5     1
## 10 2011-09-04 2011-09-05 alive  female no       15   123    83   7.2     1
## # i 203 more rows
## # i 2 more variables: stroke_type <chr>, referral_from <chr>
```

5.5.3   Rename variable using `rename()`

Now, we want to rename

- variable gender to sex
- variable ASA to asa

```
pep2 <- pep2 %>%
  rename(sex = gender,
                 asa = ASA)
```

5.6   Sorting Data and Selecting Observation

The function `arrange()` can sort the data. And the function `filter()` allows you to select observations based on your criteria.

5.6.1   Sorting data using `arrange()`

We can sort data in ascending or descending order using the `arrange()` function. For example, for dataset `stroke`, let us sort the `doa` from the earliest.

```
stroke %>%
  arrange(doa)
```

```
## # A tibble: 213 x 12
##     doa        dod        status sex    dm    gcs   sbp   dbp   wbc time2
##     <date>     <date>     <chr>  <chr>  <chr> <dbl> <dbl> <dbl> <dbl> <dbl>
##  1 2011-01-01 2011-01-05 dead   female yes      15   150    87  12.5     4
##  2 2011-01-03 2011-01-06 alive  male   no       15   152   108   7.4     3
##  3 2011-01-06 2011-01-22 alive  female yes      15   231   117  22.4    16
##  4 2011-01-16 2011-02-08 alive  female no       11   110    79   9.6    23
##  5 2011-01-18 2011-01-23 alive  male   no       15   199   134  18.7     5
##  6 2011-01-20 2011-01-24 dead   female no        7   190   101  11.3     4
##  7 2011-01-25 2011-02-16 alive  female yes       5   145   102  15.8    22
##  8 2011-01-28 2011-02-11 dead   female yes      13   161    96   8.5    14
##  9 2011-01-29 2011-02-02 alive  male   no       15   222   129   9       4
## 10 2011-01-31 2011-02-02 alive  male   no       15   161   107   9.5     2
## # i 203 more rows
## # i 2 more variables: stroke_type <chr>, referral_from <chr>
```

5.6.2 Select observation using `filter()`

We use the `filter()` function to select observations based on certain criteria. Here, in this example, we will create a new dataset (which we will name as `stroke_m_40`) that contains patients that have sex as male and Glasgow Coma Scale (gcs) at 7 or higher:

- gender is male
- gcs at 7 or higher

```
stroke_m_7 <- stroke %>%
  filter(sex == 'male', gcs >= 7)
stroke_m_7
```

```
## # A tibble: 85 x 12
##    doa        dod        status sex    dm     gcs   sbp   dbp   wbc time2
##    <date>     <date>     <chr>  <chr> <chr> <dbl> <dbl> <dbl> <dbl> <dbl>
##  1 2011-02-17 2011-02-18 alive  male  no       15   151    73  12.5     1
##  2 2011-03-20 2011-03-21 alive  male  no       15   196   123   8.1     1
##  3 2011-05-22 2011-05-23 alive  male  no       11   171    80   8.7     1
##  4 2011-11-28 2011-11-29 dead   male  no       10   207   128  10.8     1
##  5 2012-02-22 2012-02-23 dead   male  no        7   150    80  15.5     1
##  6 2012-03-25 2012-03-26 alive  male  no       14   128    79  10.3     1
##  7 2012-04-02 2012-04-03 alive  male  no       15   143    59   7.1     1
##  8 2011-01-31 2011-02-02 alive  male  no       15   161   107   9.5     2
##  9 2011-02-06 2011-02-08 alive  male  no       15   153    61  11.2     2
## 10 2011-02-20 2011-02-22 alive  male  no       15   143    93  15.6     2
## # i 75 more rows
## # i 2 more variables: stroke_type <chr>, referral_from <chr>
```

Next, we will create a new dataset (named `stroke_high_BP`) that contain

- sbp above 130 OR dbp above 90

```
stroke_high_BP <- stroke %>%
  filter(sbp > 130 | dbp > 90)
stroke_high_BP
```

```
## # A tibble: 173 x 12
##    doa        dod        status sex     dm     gcs   sbp   dbp   wbc time2
##    <date>     <date>     <chr>  <chr>  <chr> <dbl> <dbl> <dbl> <dbl> <dbl>
##  1 2011-02-17 2011-02-18 alive  male   no       15   151    73  12.5     1
##  2 2011-03-20 2011-03-21 alive  male   no       15   196   123   8.1     1
##  3 2011-04-12 2011-04-13 dead   male   no        3   170   103  13.9     1
##  4 2011-05-22 2011-05-23 alive  male   no       11   171    80   8.7     1
##  5 2011-07-11 2011-07-12 dead   female yes       6   170    90  10.5     1
```

```
##  6 2011-10-12 2011-10-13 alive  female no        15   144    89   5.7    1
##  7 2011-10-21 2011-10-22 alive  male   no         4   230   120  12.7    1
##  8 2011-10-26 2011-10-27 dead   female no         4   207   120  16.5    1
##  9 2011-11-28 2011-11-29 dead   male   no        10   207   128  10.8    1
## 10 2011-12-29 2011-12-30 alive  female no        12   178   100   8.8    1
## # i 163 more rows
## # i 2 more variables: stroke_type <chr>, referral_from <chr>
```

5.7   Group Data and Get Summary Statistics

The group_by() function allows us to group data based on categorical variable. Using the summarize we do summary statistics for the overall data or for groups created using group_by() function.

5.7.1   Group data using `group_by()`

The group_by function will prepare the data for group analysis. For example,

- to get summary values for mean sbp, mean dbp and mean gcs
- for sex

```
stroke_sex <- stroke %>%
  group_by(sex)
```

5.7.2   Summary statistic using `summarize()`

Now that we have a group data named stroke_sex, now, we would summarize our data using the mean and standard deviation (SD) for the groups specified above.

```
stroke_sex %>%
  summarise(meansbp = mean(sbp, na.rm = TRUE),
            meandbp = mean(dbp, na.rm = TRUE),
            meangcs = mean(gcs, na.rm = TRUE))
```

```
## # A tibble: 2 x 4
##   sex      meansbp meandbp meangcs
##   <chr>      <dbl>   <dbl>   <dbl>
## 1 female      166.    91.5    11.9
## 2 male        159.    91.6    13.3
```

To calculate the frequencies for two variables for pep dataset

- sex
- outcome

```
pep2 %>%
  group_by(sex) %>%
  count(outcome, sort = TRUE)
```

```
## # A tibble: 4 x 3
## # Groups:   sex [2]
##   sex     outcome      n
##   <chr>   <chr>    <int>
## 1 male    alive       70
## 2 male    dead        26
## 3 female  alive       13
## 4 female  dead        12
```

or

```
pep2 %>%
  count(sex, outcome, sort = TRUE)
```

```
##       sex outcome  n
## 1    male   alive 70
## 2    male    dead 26
## 3  female   alive 13
## 4  female    dead 12
```

5.8 More Complicated dplyr Verbs

To be more efficient, use multiple **dplyr** (a package inside tidyverse meta-package) functions in one line of R code. For example,

```
pep2 %>%
  filter(sex == "male", diastolic >= 60, systolic >= 80) %>%
  dplyr::select(age, systolic, diastolic, perforation, outcome) %>%
  group_by(outcome) %>%
  summarize(mean_sbp = mean(systolic, na.rm = TRUE),
            mean_dbp = mean(diastolic, na.rm = TRUE),
            mean_perf = mean(perforation, na.rm = TRUE),
            freq = n())
```

```
## # A tibble: 2 x 5
##   outcome mean_sbp mean_dbp mean_perf  freq
##   <chr>      <dbl>    <dbl>     <dbl> <int>
## 1 alive       135.     77.2     0.920    61
## 2 dead        130.     75.5     1.80     23
```

5.9   Data Transformation for Categorical Variables

5.9.1   forcats package

Data transformation for categorical variables (factor variables) can be facilitated using the **forcats** package.

5.9.2   Conversion from numeric to factor variables

Now, we will convert the integer (numerical) variable to a factor (categorical) variable. For example, we will generate a new factor (categorical) variable named high_bp from variables sbp and dbp (both double variables). We will label high_bp as *High* or *Not High*.

The criteria:

• if sbp $sbp \geq 130$ or $dbp \geq 90$ then labeled as High, else is Not High

```
stroke <- stroke %>%
  mutate(high_bp = if_else(sbp >= 130 | dbp >= 90,
                           "High", "Not High"))
stroke %>% count(high_bp)
```

```
## # A tibble: 2 x 2
##   high_bp      n
##   <chr>    <int>
## 1 High       177
## 2 Not High    36
```

alternatively, you can use cut()

```
stroke <- stroke %>%
  mutate(cat_sbp = cut(sbp, breaks = c(-Inf, 120, 130, Inf),
                       labels = c('<120', '121-130', '>130')))
stroke %>% count(cat_sbp)
```

```
## # A tibble: 3 x 2
```

```
##    cat_sbp      n
##    <fct>      <int>
## 1 <120          25
## 2 121-130       16
## 3 >130         172


stroke %>%
  group_by(cat_sbp) %>%
  summarize(minsbp = min(sbp),
            maxsbp = max(sbp))


## # A tibble: 3 x 3
##    cat_sbp minsbp maxsbp
##    <fct>    <dbl>  <dbl>
## 1 <120        75    120
## 2 121-130    122    130
## 3 >130       132    290
```

5.9.3   Recoding variables

We use this function to recode variables from old to new levels. For example:

```
stroke <- stroke %>%
  mutate(cat_sbp2 = recode(cat_sbp, "<120" = "120 or less",
                           "121-130" = "121 to 130",
                           ">130" = "131 or higher"))
stroke %>% count(cat_sbp2)


## # A tibble: 3 x 2
##    cat_sbp2        n
##    <fct>        <int>
## 1 120 or less     25
## 2 121 to 130      16
## 3 131 or higher  172
```

5.9.4   Changing the level of categorical variable

Variable `cat_sbp` will be ordered as

- less or 120, then
- 121 - 130, then
- 131 or higher

```
levels(stroke$cat_sbp)
```

```
## [1] "<120"     "121-130" ">130"
```

```
stroke %>% count(cat_sbp)
```

```
## # A tibble: 3 x 2
##   cat_sbp       n
##   <fct>      <int>
## 1 <120          25
## 2 121-130       16
## 3 >130         172
```

To change the order (in reverse for example), we can use fct_relevel. Below the first level group is sbp above 130, followed by 121 to 130 and the highest group is less than 120.

```
stroke <- stroke %>%
  mutate(relevel_cat_sbp = fct_relevel(cat_sbp, ">130", "121-130", "<120"))
levels(stroke$relevel_cat_sbp)
```

```
## [1] ">130"    "121-130" "<120"
```

```
stroke %>% count(relevel_cat_sbp)
```

```
## # A tibble: 3 x 2
##   relevel_cat_sbp       n
##   <fct>             <int>
## 1 >130                172
## 2 121-130              16
## 3 <120                 25
```

5.10 Additional Resources

The link to webpages below helps readers explore more about Data transformation or wrangling using R.

- **dplyr** vignettes[3]

---

[3]https://cran.r-project.org/web/packages/dplyr/vignettes/dplyr.html

- example of using **forcats** here[4]
- **rio** package[5] to help readers read data into R

5.11   Summary

dplyr package is a very useful package that encourages users to use proper verb when manipulating variables (columns) and observations (rows). We have learned to use five functions but there are more functions available. Other useful functions include `dplyr::distinct()`, `dplyr::transmutate()`, `dplyr::sample_n()` and `dplyr::sample_frac()`. If you are working with a database, you can use **dbplyr**, which performs data wrangling very effectively with databases. For categorical variables, you can use **forcats** package.

---

[4]http://r4ds.had.co.nz/factors.html
[5]https://cran.r-project.org/web/packages/rio/vignettes/rio.html

6

Exploratory Data Analysis

6.1 Objectives

At the end of the chapter, readers will be able to

- perform exploratory data analysis (EDA) using graphical methods
- perform EDA using descriptive statistics
- acquire basic skills to use **ggplot2** and **gtsummary** packages

6.2 Introduction

Exploratory Data Analysis or EDA is the critical process of performing initial investigations on data to discover patterns, spot anomalies, test hypotheses and check assumptions with the help of summary statistics and graphical representations.

In statistics, exploratory data analysis (EDA) is an approach to data analysis to summarize their main characteristics, often with visual methods. A statistical model can be used or not, but primarily EDA is for seeing what the data can tell us beyond the formal modeling or hypothesis testing task.

Exploratory data analysis was promoted by John Tukey to encourage statisticians to explore the data and possibly formulate hypotheses that could lead to new data collection (Source[1])

---

[1]https://en.wikipedia.org/wiki/Exploratory_data_analysis

DOI: 10.1201/9781003296775-6

6.3 EDA Using ggplot2 Package

6.3.1 Usage of ggplot2

We always start with `ggplot()` function, the state the specific dataset. Next, we choose the aesthetic mapping (with `aes()`) represent the variable or variables to plot) and then we add on layers. These can be converted to R codes as below:

- geom_X : `geom_point()`, `geom_histogram()`
- scales (like `scale_colour_brewer()`)
- faceting specifications (like `facet_wrap()`)
- coordinate systems (like `coord_flip()`).

6.4 Preparation

6.4.1 Load the libraries

We will use these packages for data exploration:

1. **tidyverse** package for plotting and data wrangling
2. **gtsummary** package for summary statistics
3. **patchwork** to combine plots
4. **here** to point to the correct working directory
5. **readxl** to read a MS Excel file

The tidyverse is an opinionated collection of R packages designed for data science. All packages share an underlying design philosophy, grammar, and data structures. We may find more information about the package here[2]

```
library(tidyverse)
```

```
## -- Attaching core tidyverse packages ----------------------- tidyverse 2.0.0 -
-
## v dplyr     1.1.1     v readr     2.1.4
## v forcats   1.0.0     v stringr   1.5.0
## v ggplot2   3.4.2     v tibble    3.2.1
## v lubridate 1.9.2     v tidyr     1.3.0
## v purrr     1.0.1
```

---

[2]https://www.tidyverse.org/

```
##            --         Conflicts        -----------------------------------------
tidyverse_conflicts() --
## x dplyr::filter() masks stats::filter()
## x dplyr::lag()    masks stats::lag()
##    i   Use    the    conflicted    package    (<http://conflicted.r-
lib.org/>) to force all conflicts to become errors
```

```
library(gtsummary)
library(patchwork)
library(here)
```

```
## here() starts at C:/Users/drkim/Downloads/multivar_data_analysis/multivar_data_analysis
```

```
library(readxl)
```

6.4.2 Read the dataset into R

Let us read the *peptic ulcer data* in MS Excel format. To do this, we will

- load the **readxl** package
- use the function `read_xlsx()` to read data into R

```
pep <- read_xlsx(here('data', 'peptic_ulcer.xlsx'))
```

Examine the data by looking a the number of observations, type of variables and name of variables.

```
glimpse(pep)
```

```
## Rows: 121
## Columns: 34
## $ age                <dbl> 42, 66, 67, 19, 77, 39, 62, 71, 69, 97, 52, 21, 57~
## $ gender             <chr> "male", "female", "male", "male", "male", "male", ~
## $ epigastric_pain    <chr> "yes", "yes", "yes", "yes", "yes", "yes", "yes", "~
## $ vomiting           <chr> "no", "no", "no", "no", "yes", "no", "no", "yes", ~
## $ nausea             <chr> "no", "no", "no", "no", "yes", "no", "no", "no", "~
## $ fever              <chr> "no", "no", "no", "no", "no", "yes", "no", "yes", ~
## $ diarrhea           <chr> "no", "no", "yes", "no", "no", "no", "no", "yes", ~
## $ malena             <chr> "no", "no", "no", "no", "no", "no", "no", "no", "n~
## $ onset_more_24_hrs  <chr> "no", "no", "no", "yes", "yes", "yes", "yes", "no"~
## $ NSAIDS             <chr> "no", "no", "yes", "no", "no", "no", "no", "no", "~
## $ septic_shock       <chr> "no", "no", "no", "no", "no", "no", "no", "no", "n~
```

```
## $ previous_OGDS   <chr> "no", "no", "no", "yes", "no", "no", "no", "no", "~
## $ ASA             <dbl> 1, 1, 1, 1, 2, 1, 2, 2, 1, 1, 2, 1, 2, 1, 1, 2, 2,~
## $ systolic        <dbl> 141, 197, 126, 90, 147, 115, 103, 159, 145, 105, 1~
## $ diastolic       <dbl> 98, 88, 73, 40, 82, 86, 55, 68, 75, 65, 74, 50, 86~
## $ inotropes       <chr> "no", "no", "no", "no", "no", "no", "no", "no", "n~
## $ pulse           <dbl> 109, 126, 64, 112, 89, 96, 100, 57, 86, 100, 109, ~
## $ tenderness      <chr> "generalized", "generalized", "generalized", "loca~
## $ guarding        <chr> "yes", "yes", "yes", "yes", "no", "yes", "yes", "n~
## $ hemoglobin      <dbl> 18.0, 12.0, 12.0, 12.0, 11.0, 18.0, 8.1, 13.3, 11.~
## $ twc             <dbl> 6.0, 6.0, 13.0, 20.0, 21.0, 4.0, 5.0, 12.0, 6.0, 2~
## $ platelet        <dbl> 415, 292, 201, 432, 324, 260, 461, 210, 293, 592, ~
## $ creatinine      <dbl> 135, 66, 80, 64, 137, 102, 69, 92, 94, 104, 58, 24~
## $ albumin         <chr> "27", "28", "32", "42", "38", "38", "30", "41", "N~
## $ PULP            <dbl> 2, 3, 3, 2, 7, 1, 2, 5, 3, 4, 2, 3, 4, 3, 5, 5, 1,~
## $ admission_to_op_hrs <dbl> 2, 2, 3, 3, 3, 3, 4, 4, 4, 4, 4, 5, 5, 6, 6, 6, 6,~
## $ perforation     <dbl> 0.5, 1.0, 0.5, 0.5, 1.0, 1.0, 3.0, 1.5, 0.5, 1.5, ~
## $ degree_perforation <chr> "small", "small", "small", "small", "small", "smal~
## $ side_perforation   <chr> "distal stomach", "distal stomach", "distal stomac~
## $ ICU             <chr> "no", "no", "no", "no", "yes", "no", "yes", "no", ~
## $ SSSI            <chr> "no", "no", "no", "no", "no", "no", "no", "no", "n~
## $ anast_leak      <chr> "no", "no", "no", "no", "no", "no", "no", "no", "n~
## $ sepsis          <chr> "no", "no", "no", "no", "no", "no", "yes", "no", "~
## $ outcome         <chr> "alive", "alive", "alive", "alive", "alive", "aliv~
```

The are quite several variables. For the sake of simplicity, we will select variables which we think might be important for simple data exploration using the `select()` function.

```
pep <- pep %>%
  select(age, systolic, diastolic, hemoglobin, twc,
         ASA, PULP, perforation, gender, epigastric_pain,
         malena, tenderness, degree_perforation, outcome)
```

6.5   EDA in Tables

We can get the overall descriptive statistics for the peptic ulcer data by using the `tbl_summary` function.

```
pep %>%
  tbl_summary(
```

```
    statistic = list(all_continuous() ~ "{mean} ({sd})",
                     all_categorical() ~ "{n} / {N} ({p}%)"),
    digits = all_continuous() ~ 2) %>%
  modify_caption("Patient Characteristics (N = {N})") %>%
  as_gt()
```

Characteristic	N = 121[1]
age	60.43 (18.05)
systolic	128.56 (24.51)
diastolic	72.07 (13.99)
hemoglobin	12.32 (3.33)
twc	13.03 (6.66)
ASA	
1	63 / 121 (52%)
2	50 / 121 (41%)
3	8 / 121 (6.6%)
PULP	3.53 (2.28)
perforation	1.22 (0.91)
gender	
female	25 / 121 (21%)
male	96 / 121 (79%)
epigastric_pain	116 / 121 (96%)
malena	4 / 121 (3.3%)
tenderness	
generalized	84 / 121 (69%)
localized	37 / 121 (31%)
degree_perforation	
large	26 / 121 (21%)
moderate	20 / 121 (17%)
small	75 / 121 (62%)
outcome	
alive	83 / 121 (69%)
dead	38 / 121 (31%)

[1]Mean (SD); n / N (%)

To stratify the descriptive statistics based on variable outcome, we use the argument
`by =`.

```
tab_outcome <- pep %>%
  tbl_summary(
    by = outcome,
```

```
  statistic = list(all_continuous() ~ "{mean} ({sd})",
                   all_categorical() ~ "{n} / {N} ({p}%)"),
  digits = all_continuous() ~ 2) %>%
modify_caption("Patient Characteristics and Fatality (N = {N})")

tab_outcome %>%
  as_gt()
```

Characteristic	**alive**, N = 83[1]	**dead**, N = 38[1]
age	58.20 (18.53)	65.29 (16.14)
systolic	130.95 (25.06)	123.34 (22.71)
diastolic	73.25 (14.02)	69.50 (13.75)
hemoglobin	12.74 (3.14)	11.41 (3.57)
twc	12.75 (6.00)	13.64 (7.96)
ASA		
1	49 / 83 (59%)	14 / 38 (37%)
2	28 / 83 (34%)	22 / 38 (58%)
3	6 / 83 (7.2%)	2 / 38 (5.3%)
PULP	3.16 (2.35)	4.34 (1.89)
perforation	0.95 (0.60)	1.82 (1.16)
gender		
female	13 / 83 (16%)	12 / 38 (32%)
male	70 / 83 (84%)	26 / 38 (68%)
epigastric_pain	79 / 83 (95%)	37 / 38 (97%)
malena	2 / 83 (2.4%)	2 / 38 (5.3%)
tenderness		
generalized	60 / 83 (72%)	24 / 38 (63%)
localized	23 / 83 (28%)	14 / 38 (37%)
degree_perforation		
large	9 / 83 (11%)	17 / 38 (45%)
moderate	13 / 83 (16%)	7 / 38 (18%)
small	61 / 83 (73%)	14 / 38 (37%)

[1]Mean (SD); n / N (%)

Next, we stratify the descriptive statistics based on gender also using the by = argument.

```
tab_gender <- pep %>%
  tbl_summary(
    by = gender,
    statistic = list(all_continuous() ~ "{mean} ({sd})",
```

```
                   all_categorical() ~ "{n} / {N} ({p}%)"),
    digits = all_continuous() ~ 2) %>%
  modify_caption("**Patient Characteristics and Gender** (N = {N})")

tab_gender %>%
  as_gt()
```

Characteristic	**female**, N = 25[1]	**male**, N = 96[1]
age	70.12 (11.07)	57.91 (18.70)
systolic	125.84 (26.17)	129.27 (24.16)
diastolic	66.68 (13.57)	73.48 (13.82)
hemoglobin	10.43 (3.09)	12.81 (3.22)
twc	11.06 (7.44)	13.54 (6.38)
ASA		
1	13 / 25 (52%)	50 / 96 (52%)
2	11 / 25 (44%)	39 / 96 (41%)
3	1 / 25 (4.0%)	7 / 96 (7.3%)
PULP	4.32 (1.86)	3.32 (2.34)
perforation	1.49 (1.14)	1.16 (0.83)
epigastric_pain	24 / 25 (96%)	92 / 96 (96%)
malena	1 / 25 (4.0%)	3 / 96 (3.1%)
tenderness		
generalized	17 / 25 (68%)	67 / 96 (70%)
localized	8 / 25 (32%)	29 / 96 (30%)
degree_perforation		
large	7 / 25 (28%)	19 / 96 (20%)
moderate	4 / 25 (16%)	16 / 96 (17%)
small	14 / 25 (56%)	61 / 96 (64%)
outcome		
alive	13 / 25 (52%)	70 / 96 (73%)
dead	12 / 25 (48%)	26 / 96 (27%)

[1]Mean (SD); n / N (%)

We can combine the two tables using `tbl_merge()`.

```
tbl_merge(
  tbls = list(tab_gender, tab_outcome),
  tab_spanner = c("**Gender**", "**Outcome**")) %>%
  as_gt()
```

Characteristic	Gender		Outcome	
	female, N = 25[1]	**male**, N = 96[1]	**alive**, N = 83[1]	**dead**, N = 38[1]
age	70.12 (11.07)	57.91 (18.70)	58.20 (18.53)	65.29 (16.14)
systolic	125.84 (26.17)	129.27 (24.16)	130.95 (25.06)	123.34 (22.71)
diastolic	66.68 (13.57)	73.48 (13.82)	73.25 (14.02)	69.50 (13.75)
hemoglobin	10.43 (3.09)	12.81 (3.22)	12.74 (3.14)	11.41 (3.57)
twc	11.06 (7.44)	13.54 (6.38)	12.75 (6.00)	13.64 (7.96)
ASA				
1	13 / 25 (52%)	50 / 96 (52%)	49 / 83 (59%)	14 / 38 (37%)
2	11 / 25 (44%)	39 / 96 (41%)	28 / 83 (34%)	22 / 38 (58%)
3	1 / 25 (4.0%)	7 / 96 (7.3%)	6 / 83 (7.2%)	2 / 38 (5.3%)
PULP	4.32 (1.86)	3.32 (2.34)	3.16 (2.35)	4.34 (1.89)
perforation	1.49 (1.14)	1.16 (0.83)	0.95 (0.60)	1.82 (1.16)
epigastric_pain	24 / 25 (96%)	92 / 96 (96%)	79 / 83 (95%)	37 / 38 (97%)
malena	1 / 25 (4.0%)	3 / 96 (3.1%)	2 / 83 (2.4%)	2 / 38 (5.3%)
tenderness				
generalized	17 / 25 (68%)	67 / 96 (70%)	60 / 83 (72%)	24 / 38 (63%)
localized	8 / 25 (32%)	29 / 96 (30%)	23 / 83 (28%)	14 / 38 (37%)
degree_perforation				
large	7 / 25 (28%)	19 / 96 (20%)	9 / 83 (11%)	17 / 38 (45%)
moderate	4 / 25 (16%)	16 / 96 (17%)	13 / 83 (16%)	7 / 38 (18%)
small	14 / 25 (56%)	61 / 96 (64%)	61 / 83 (73%)	14 / 38 (37%)
outcome				
alive	13 / 25 (52%)	70 / 96 (73%)		
dead	12 / 25 (48%)	26 / 96 (27%)		
gender				
female			13 / 83 (16%)	12 / 38 (32%)
male			70 / 83 (84%)	26 / 38 (68%)

[1]Mean (SD); n / N (%)

6.6 EDA with Plots

6.6.1 One variable: Distribution of a categorical variable

6.6.1.1 Bar chart

The frequency of the outcome

```
pep %>%
  group_by(outcome) %>%
  summarise(freq = n())
```

```
## # A tibble: 2 x 2
##    outcome  freq
##    <chr>    <int>
## 1 alive       83
## 2 dead        38
```

To plot the distribution of a categorical variable, we can use a Bar chart.

```
ggplot(data = pep) +
  geom_bar(mapping = aes(x = outcome)) +
  theme_bw()
```

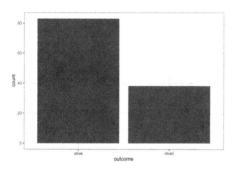

But we can also pass the aes() to ggplot

```
ggplot(data = pep, mapping = aes(x = outcome)) +
  geom_bar() +
  theme_bw()
```

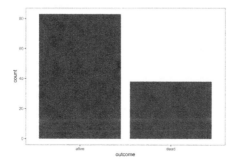

Readers can combine **dplyr** for data wrangling and then **ggplot2** (both are packages inside the **tidyverse** metapackage) to plot the data. For example, **dplyr** part for data wrangling:

```
pep_age <- pep %>% group_by(outcome) %>%
  summarize(mean_age = mean(age))
pep_age
```

```
## # A tibble: 2 x 2
##    outcome mean_age
##    <chr>      <dbl>
## 1 alive       58.2
## 2 dead        65.3
```

And the **ggplot2** part to make the plot:

```
ggplot(pep_age, mapping = aes(x = outcome, y = mean_age)) +
  geom_col()
```

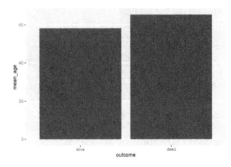

We can combine both tasks **dplyr** and **ggplot** together that will save time:

```
pep %>%
  group_by(outcome) %>%
  summarize(mean_age = mean(age)) %>%
  ggplot(mapping = aes(x = outcome, y = mean_age, fill = outcome)) +
  geom_col() +
  ylab("Mean age (Years)") +
  xlab("Outcome of ulcer") +
  scale_fill_grey() +
  theme_bw()
```

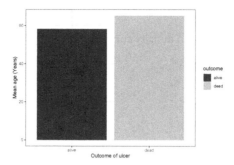

As we mentioned before, an excellent resource for graphics using **ggplot2** is availble on this website[3]. It is a must-go-to website. Of if you prefer the read the physical version, purchase the R Graphics Cookbook (Chang, 2013).

6.6.2 One variable: Distribution of a numerical variable

6.6.2.1 Histogram

To plot the distribution of a numerical variable, we can plot a histogram. To specify the number of bin, we can use binwidth and add some customization.

```
ggplot(data = pep, mapping = aes(x = systolic)) +
  geom_histogram(binwidth = 10) +
  ylab("Frequency") +
  xlab("Systolic Blood Pressure") +
  ggtitle("Systolic BP distribution") +
  theme_bw()
```

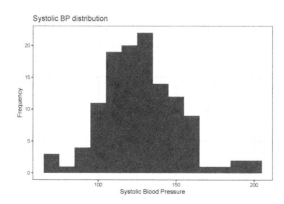

---

[3]http://www.cookbook-r.com/Graphs/Bar_and_line_graphs_(ggplot2)/

6.6.2.2   Density curve

Let us create a density curve. A density curve also helps us examine the distribution of observations.

```
ggplot(data = pep, mapping = aes(x = diastolic)) +
  geom_density() +
  xlab("Diastolic BP (mmHg)") +
  ylab("Density") +
  labs(title = "Density distribution for diastolic BP",
       caption = "Source : Peptic ulcer disease data") +
  theme_bw()
```

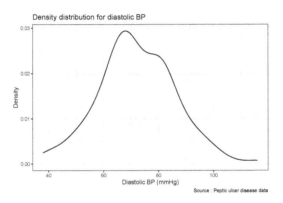

6.6.2.3   Histogram and density curve together

If we want to plot both the histogram and the density curve, we can use `geom_histogram()` and `geom_density()` in the single line of codes, we can combine two geoms.

```
ggplot(pep, mapping = aes(x = diastolic)) +
  geom_histogram(mapping = aes(y = ..density..), binwidth = 10) +
  geom_density() +
  xlab("Diastolic BP (mmHg)") +
  ylab("Density") +
  labs(title = "Density distribution for diastolic BP",
       caption = "Source : Peptic ulcer disease data") +
  theme_bw()
```

```
## Warning: The dot-dot notation (`..density..`) was deprecated in ggplot2 3.4.0.
## i Please use `after_stat(density)` instead.
## This warning is displayed once every 8 hours.
```

```
## Call `lifecycle::last_lifecycle_warnings()` to see where this warning was
## generated.
```

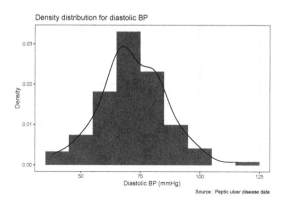

6.6.3   Two variables: Plotting a numerical and a categorical variable

6.6.3.1   Overlaying histograms and boxplot

By overlaying histograms, examine the distribution of a numerical variable (var **age**) based on variable **outcome**. First, we create an object called hist_age. Next, we create a boxplot object and name it as box-age. After that, we combine the two objects side-by-side using a vertical bar.

```
hist_age <- ggplot(data = pep, aes(x = age, fill = outcome)) +
  geom_histogram(binwidth = 5, aes(y = ..density..),
                 position = "identity", alpha = 0.75) +
  geom_density(alpha = 0.25) +
  xlab("Age") +
  ylab("Density") +
  labs(title = "Density distribution",
       caption = "Source : Peptic ulcer disease data") +
    scale_fill_grey() +
  theme_bw()


box_age <- ggplot(data = pep, aes(x = outcome, y = age)) +
  geom_boxplot(outlier.shape = NA) +
  geom_dotplot(binaxis = "y", binwidth = 1, fill = NA,
               alpha = 0.85) +
  xlab('Outcome') + ylab('Age') +
```

```
labs(title = "Box-plot",
     caption = "Source : Peptic ulcer disease data") +
theme_bw()
```

When we plot using Rmarkdown, we set the width of the figure as 9 and height as 4 *r* *,fig.width=9, fig.height=4* in the R code chunk to better show the plots side by side. And then set the width of the figure as 9 and height as 4 *r,fig.width=9, fig.height=4* for the plots in vertical arrangement.You can read more placement of multiple plots from the **patchwork** package[4] to learn about arranging multiple plots in a single figure.

```
hist_age  |  box_age
```

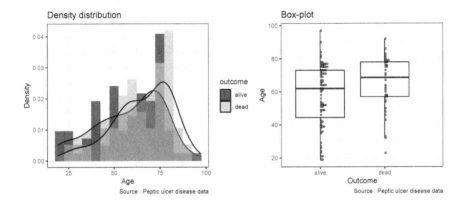

```
hist_age  /  box_age
```

---

[4]https://patchwork.data-imaginist.com/

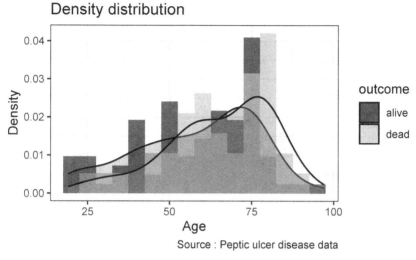

Source : Peptic ulcer disease data

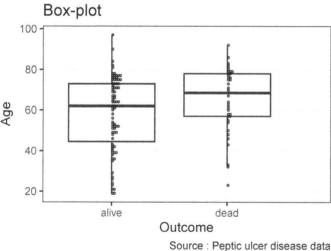

Source : Peptic ulcer disease data

6.6.4   Three variables: Plotting a numerical and two categorical variables

It is hard to visualize three variables in a single histogram plot. But we can use `facet_.()` function to further split the plots.

6.6.5   Faceting the plots

We can see better plots if we split the histogram based on a particular grouping. In this example, we stratify the distribution of variable age (a numerical variable) based on outcome and gender (both are categorical variables)

```r
ggplot(data = pep, aes(x = age, fill = gender)) +
    geom_histogram(binwidth = 5, aes(y = ..density..),
                    position = "identity", alpha = 0.45) +
  geom_density(aes(linetype = gender), alpha = 0.65) +
  scale_fill_grey() +
  xlab("Age") +
  ylab("Density") +
  labs(title = "Density distribution of age for outcome and gender",
        caption = "Source : Peptic ulcer disease data") +
  theme_bw() +
  facet_wrap( ~ outcome)
```

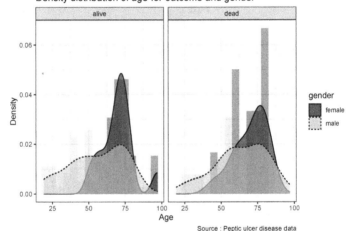

We can provide the summary statistics to complement the plots or vice versa.

```r
pep %>%
  group_by(outcome, gender) %>%
  summarize(mean_age = mean(age, na.rm = TRUE),
            sd_age = sd(age, na.rm = TRUE))
```

```
## `summarise()` has grouped output by 'outcome'. You can override using the
## `.groups` argument.

## # A tibble: 4 x 4
## # Groups:   outcome [2]
##    outcome gender mean_age sd_age
##    <chr>   <chr>     <dbl>  <dbl>
```

```
## 1 alive    female    70.2    11.4
## 2 alive    male      56.0    18.8
## 3 dead     female    70.1    11.2
## 4 dead     male      63.1    17.7
```

6.6.6 Line plot

Line graphs are typically used for visualizing how one continuous variable on the y-axis changes concerning another continuous variable on the x-axis. This is very useful for longitudinal data. Line graphs can also be used with a discrete variable on the x-axis. This is appropriate when the variable is ordered (e.g. "small", "medium", and "large").

Let us Load **gapminder** package and view the variables and the observations of the *gapminder* dataset.

```
library(gapminder)
glimpse(gapminder)
```

```
## Rows: 1,704
## Columns: 6
## $ country   <fct> "Afghanistan", "Afghanistan", "Afghanistan", "Afghanistan", ~
## $ continent <fct> Asia, Asia, Asia, Asia, Asia, Asia, Asia, Asia, Asia, Asia, ~
## $ year      <int> 1952, 1957, 1962, 1967, 1972, 1977, 1982, 1987, 1992, 1997, ~
## $ lifeExp   <dbl> 28.801, 30.332, 31.997, 34.020, 36.088, 38.438, 39.854, 40.8~
## $ pop       <int> 8425333, 9240934, 10267083, 11537966, 13079460, 14880372, 12~
## $ gdpPercap <dbl> 779.4453, 820.8530, 853.1007, 836.1971, 739.9811, 786.1134, ~
```

We can plot the relationship between variable life expectancy `lifeExp` only for countried in the Asia continent. To do so, we

- specify the data. In this case the *gapminder* dataset
- choose only Asia continent using the `filter()`
- choose variable life expectancy for the y axis and year for the x axis. Then we will give different lines to represent different countries.
- will use `geom_line()` to generate the line plot

```
gapminder %>%
  filter(continent == "Asia") %>%
  ggplot(mapping = aes(x = year, y = lifeExp, linetype = country)) +
  geom_line(show.legend = FALSE) +
  xlab("Year") + ylab("Life Expectancy") +
  theme_bw()
```

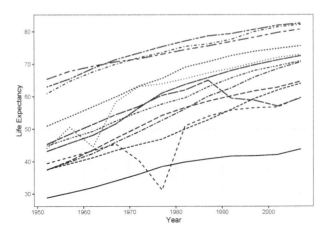

And the summary statistics for the plot.

```
gapminder %>%
  filter(continent == 'Asia') %>%
  filter(year == 1962 | year == 1982 | year == 2002) %>%
  group_by(year) %>%
  summarise(mean_life = mean(lifeExp, na.rm = TRUE),
            sd_life = sd(lifeExp, na.rm = TRUE))
```

```
## # A tibble: 3 x 3
##     year mean_life sd_life
##    <int>     <dbl>   <dbl>
## 1   1962      51.6    9.82
## 2   1982      62.6    8.54
## 3   2002      69.2    8.37
```

We may use **gtsummary** package to generate publication ready table. We need to filter for Asia continent only to represent the line plot we generated before.

```
gapminder %>%
  select(continent, year, lifeExp, pop, gdpPercap) %>%
  filter(continent == "Asia") %>%
  filter(year == 1962 | year == 1982 | year == 2002) %>%
  mutate(pop = pop/1000000, gdpPercap = gdpPercap/1000) %>%
  tbl_strata(
    strata = continent,
    .tbl_fun =
      ~.x %>%
      tbl_summary(
```

```
      by = year,
      label = list(lifeExp ~ "Life Exp", pop ~ "Pop size", gdpPercap ~ "Percap
      ↪  GDP"),
      statistic = list(all_continuous() ~ "{mean} ({sd})",
                       all_categorical() ~ "{n} / {N} ({p}%)"),
      missing = "no",
      digits = all_continuous() ~ 1
      )) %>%
  modify_footnote(all_stat_cols() ~ "Mean(SD), Pop size in million and GDP in
  ↪  thousand") %>%
  as_gt()
```

Characteristic	Asia		
	1962, N = 33[1]	**1982**, N = 33[1]	**2002**, N = 33[1]
Life Exp	51.6 (9.8)	62.6 (8.5)	69.2 (8.4)
Pop size	51.4 (136.1)	79.1 (206.5)	109.1 (276.7)
Percap GDP	5.7 (16.4)	7.4 (8.7)	10.2 (11.2)

[1]Mean(SD), Pop size in million and GDP in thousand

6.6.7   Plotting means and error bars

We want to error bar for life expectancy for Asia continent only. Error bar that contains mean and standard deviation

Our approach is use filter to choose Asia continent only `filter()`. Then generate the mean and SD for life expectancy using `mutate()`. Next is to plot the scatterplot (country vs mean life expectancy) `geom_point()` and then plot errorbar `geom_errorbar()`

```
gap_continent <- gapminder %>%
  filter(continent == "Asia") %>%
  group_by(country) %>%
  mutate(mean = mean(lifeExp), sd = sd(lifeExp)) %>%
  arrange(desc(mean))
```

Plot them with `coord_flip()` and use the black and white theme. We also set `fig.width=5`, `fig.height=8` in the R code chuck.

```
gap_continent %>%
  ggplot(mapping = aes(x = country, y = mean)) +
  geom_point(mapping = aes(x = country, y = mean)) +
```

```
geom_errorbar(mapping = aes(ymin = mean - sd, ymax = mean + sd),
              position = position_dodge()) +
coord_flip() +
theme_bw()
```

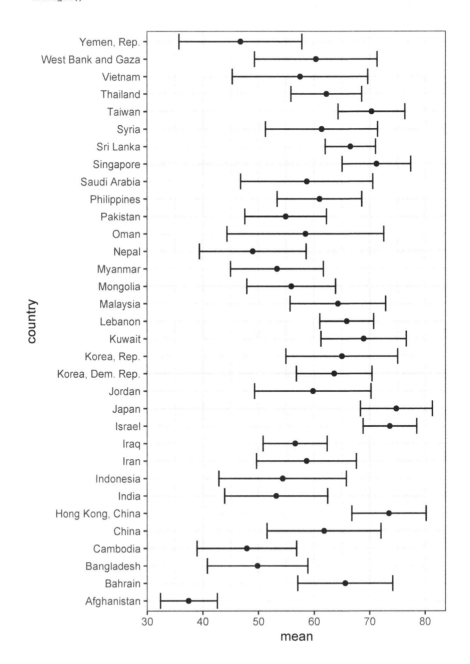

6.6.8 Scatterplot with fit line

We are using the peptic ulcer data `pep` where we will create a fit line between age and size of perforation. We then plot the scatterplot and a fit line on it. We name the plot object generated as `pep_fit`.

```
pep_fit <- pep %>%
  ggplot(aes(x = age, y = perforation, shape = outcome)) +
  geom_point(show.legend = TRUE) +
  geom_smooth(aes(x = age, y = perforation, linetype = outcome),
                  method = lm, se = FALSE) +
  ylab('Size of perforation') +
  xlab('Age of patient') +
  labs(title = 'Distribution and fit line',
       caption = 'Source: Peptic ulcer data') +
  theme_bw()
pep_fit
```

```
## `geom_smooth()` using formula = 'y ~ x'
```

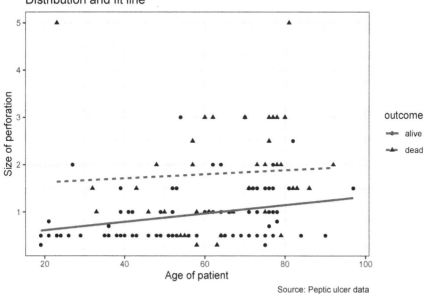

Let us see if the patterns are similar for men and women. We will use `facet_wrap()` to split the plots based on variable gender.

```
pep_fit + facet_grid(. ~ gender)
```

```
## `geom_smooth()` using formula = 'y ~ x'
```

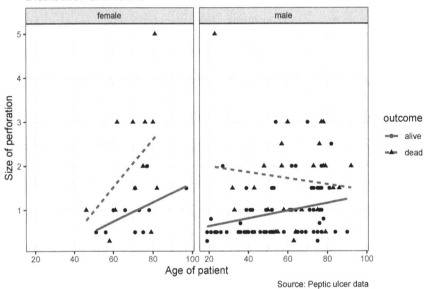

```
pep %>%
  select(gender, perforation, age) %>%
  tbl_summary(
    by = gender,
    statistic = list(all_continuous() ~ "{mean} ({sd})",
                     all_categorical() ~ "{n} / {N} ({p}%)"),
    missing = "no",
    digits = all_continuous() ~ 2 ) %>%
  modify_caption("**Patient Characteristics and Gender** (N = {N})") %>%
  as_gt()
```

Characteristic	female, N = 25[1]	male, N = 96[1]
perforation	1.49 (1.14)	1.16 (0.83)
age	70.12 (11.07)	57.91 (18.70)

[1]Mean (SD)

6.7 Summary

This chapter provides understanding to readers about exploratory data analysis (EDA) and skills to perform EDA and descriptive statistics. We learned about graphical methods in R and how to report descriptive statistics in tables. We show readers how to read an MS Excel data and then use three important packages to perform EDA (**dplyr**, **ggplot2** and **gtsummary** packages) on the data. The excellent resources available to help readers perform more complicated exploratory data analysis include *ggplot2: Elegant Graphics for Data Analysis* webpage[5] or its physical book (Chang, 2013), **ggplot2** package[6], **gtsummary** webpage[7] (Sjoberg et al., 2021) and *R for Data Science* website[8] or its physical book (Wickham and Grolemund, 2017).

---

[5] https://ggplot2-book.org/arranging-plots.html
[6] https://ggplot2.tidyverse.org/
[7] https://www.danieldsjoberg.com/gtsummary/
[8] https://r4ds.had.co.nz/

7

Linear Regression

7.1 Objectives

After completing this chapter, the readers are expected to

- understand the concept of simple and multiple linear regression
- perform simple linear regression
- perform multiple linear regression
- perform model fit assessment of linear regression models
- present and interpret the results of linear regression analyses

7.2 Introduction

Linear regression is one of the most common statistical analyses in medical and health sciences. Linear regression models the linear (i.e. straight line) relationship between:

- **outcome**: numerical variable (e.g. blood pressure, BMI and cholesterol level).
- **predictors/independent variables**: numerical variables and categorical variables (e.g. gender, race and education level).

In simple words, we might be interested in knowing the relationship between the cholesterol level and its associated factors, for example gender, age, BMI and lifestyle. This can be explored by linear regression analysis.

7.3 Linear Regression Models

Linear regression is a type of generalized linear models (GLMs), which also includes other outcome types, for example categorical and count. In subsequent chapters, we will cover these outcome types in form of logistic regression and Poisson regression.

Basically, the relationship between the outcome and predictors in linear regression is structured as follows,

$$numerical\ outcome = numerical\ predictors$$
$$+ categorical\ predictors$$

More appropriate forms of this relationship will explained later under simple and multiple linear regressions sections.

7.4   Prepare R Environment for Analysis

7.4.1   Libraries

For this chapter, we will be using the following packages:

- **foreign**: for reading SPSS and STATA datasets
- **tidyverse**: a general and powerful package for data transformation
- **psych**: for descriptive statistics
- **gtsummary**: for coming up with nice tables for results and plotting the graphs
- **ggplot2**, **ggpubr**, **GGally**: for plotting the graphs
- **rsq**: for getting R^2 value from a GLM model
- **broom**: for tidying up the results
- **car**: for `vif()` function

These are loaded as follows using the function `library()`,

```
library(foreign)
library(tidyverse)
library(psych)
library(gtsummary)
library(ggplot2)
library(ggpubr)
library(GGally)
library(rsq)
library(broom)
library(car)
```

7.4.2   Dataset

We will use the `coronary.dta` dataset in STATA format. The dataset contains the total cholesterol level, their individual characteristics and intervention groups in a hypothetical clinical trial. The dataset contains 200 observations for nine variables:

1. *id*: Subjects' ID.
2. *cad*: Coronary artery disease status (categorical) {no cad, cad}.
3. *sbp* : Systolic blood pressure in mmHg (numerical).
4. *dbp* : Diastolic blood pressure in mmHg (numerical).
5. *chol*: Total cholesterol level in mmol/L (numerical).
6. *age*: Age in years (numerical).
7. *bmi*: Body mass index (numerical).
8. *race*: Race of the subjects (categorical) {malay, chinese, indian}.
9. *gender*: Gender of the subjects (categorical) {woman, man}.

The dataset is loaded as follows,

```
coronary = read.dta("data/coronary.dta")
```

We then look at the basic structure of the dataset,

```
str(coronary)
```

```
## 'data.frame':    200 obs. of  9 variables:
## $ id     : num  1 14 56 61 62 64 69 108 112 134 ...
## $ cad    : Factor w/ 2 levels "no cad","cad": 1 1 1 1 1 1 2 1 1 1 ...
## $ sbp    : num  106 130 136 138 115 124 110 112 138 104 ...
## $ dbp    : num  68 78 84 100 85 72 80 70 85 70 ...
## $ chol   : num  6.57 6.33 5.97 7.04 6.66 ...
## $ age    : num  60 34 36 45 53 43 44 50 43 48 ...
## $ bmi    : num  38.9 37.8 40.5 37.6 40.3 ...
## $ race   : Factor w/ 3 levels "malay","chinese",..: 3 1 1 1 3 1 1 2 2 2 ...
## $ gender: Factor w/ 2 levels "woman","man": 1 1 1 1 2 2 2 1 1 2 ...
## - attr(*, "datalabel")= chr "Written by R.                    "
## - attr(*, "time.stamp")= chr ""
## - attr(*, "formats")= chr [1:9] "%9.0g" "%9.0g" "%9.0g" "%9.0g" ...
## - attr(*, "types")= int [1:9] 100 108 100 100 100 100 100 108 108
## - attr(*, "val.labels")= chr [1:9] "" "cad" "" "" ...
## - attr(*, "var.labels")= chr [1:9] "id" "cad" "sbp" "dbp" ...
## - attr(*, "version")= int 7
## - attr(*, "label.table")=List of 3
##   ..$ cad    : Named int [1:2] 1 2
##   .. ..- attr(*, "names")= chr [1:2] "no cad" "cad"
##   ..$ race   : Named int [1:3] 1 2 3
##   .. ..- attr(*, "names")= chr [1:3] "malay" "chinese" "indian"
##   ..$ gender: Named int [1:2] 1 2
##   .. ..- attr(*, "names")= chr [1:2] "woman" "man"
```

7.5   Simple Linear Regression

7.5.1   About simple linear regression

Simple linear regression (SLR) models *linear* (straight line) relationship between:

- **outcome**: numerical variable.
- **ONE predictor**: numerical/categorical variable.

Note: When the predictor is a categorical variable, this is typically analyzed by one-way ANOVA. However, SLR can also handle a categorical variable in the GLM framework.

We may formally represent SLR in form of an equation as follows,

$$numerical\ outcome = intercept + coefficient \times predictor$$

or in a shorter form using mathematical notations,

$$\hat{y} = b_0 + b_1 x_1$$

where $\hat{y}$ (pronounced y hat) is the predicted value of the outcome y.

7.5.2   Data exploration

Let say, for the SLR we are interested in knowing whether diastolic blood pressure (predictor) is associated with the cholesterol level (outcome). We explore the variables by obtaining the descriptive statistics and plotting the data distribution.

We obtain the descriptive statistics of the variables,

```
coronary %>% select(chol, dbp) %>% describe()
```

```
##         vars   n  mean    sd median trimmed   mad min    max range skew kurtosis
## chol      1 200  6.20  1.18   6.19    6.18  1.18   4   9.35  5.35 0.18    -0.31
## dbp       2 200 82.31 12.90  80.00   81.68 14.83  56 120.00 64.00 0.42    -0.33
##          se
## chol 0.08
## dbp  0.91
```

and the histograms and box-and-whiskers plots,

```
hist_chol = ggplot(coronary, aes(chol)) +
  geom_histogram(color = "black", fill = "white")
hist_dbp = ggplot(coronary, aes(dbp)) +
```

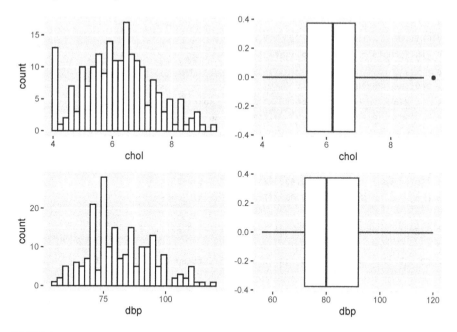

FIGURE 7.1
Histograms and box-and-whiskers plots for chol and dbp.

```
  geom_histogram(color = "black", fill = "white")
bplot_chol = ggplot(coronary, aes(chol)) +
  geom_boxplot()
bplot_dbp = ggplot(coronary, aes(dbp)) +
  geom_boxplot()
ggarrange(hist_chol, bplot_chol, hist_dbp, bplot_dbp)
```

7.5.3   Univariable analysis

For the analysis, we fit the SLR model, which consists of only one predictor (univariable). Here, chol is specified as the outcome, and dbp as the predictor. In glm, the formula is specified as outcome ~ predictor. Here, we specify chol ~ dbp as the formula in glm.

We fit and view the summary information of the model as,

```
slr_chol = glm(chol ~ dbp, data = coronary)
summary(slr_chol)
```

```
##
## Call:
## glm(formula = chol ~ dbp, data = coronary)
##
## Deviance Residuals:
##     Min       1Q   Median       3Q      Max
## -1.9967  -0.8304  -0.1292   0.7734   2.8470
##
## Coefficients:
##              Estimate Std. Error t value Pr(>|t|)
## (Intercept) 2.995134   0.492092   6.087 5.88e-09 ***
## dbp         0.038919   0.005907   6.589 3.92e-10 ***
## ---
## Signif. codes:  0 '***' 0.001 '**' 0.01 '*' 0.05 '.' 0.1 ' ' 1
##
## (Dispersion parameter for gaussian family taken to be 1.154763)
##
##      Null deviance: 278.77  on 199  degrees of freedom
## Residual deviance: 228.64  on 198  degrees of freedom
## AIC: 600.34
##
## Number of Fisher Scoring iterations: 2
```

We can tidy up the glm output and obtain the 95% confidence interval (CI) using tidy() from the broom package,

```
tidy(slr_chol, conf.int = TRUE)
```

```
## # A tibble: 2 x 7
##   term        estimate std.error statistic  p.value conf.low conf.high
##   <chr>          <dbl>     <dbl>     <dbl>    <dbl>    <dbl>     <dbl>
## 1 (Intercept)   3.00      0.492      6.09 5.88e- 9   2.03      3.96
## 2 dbp           0.0389    0.00591    6.59 3.92e-10   0.0273    0.0505
```

From the output above, we pay attention at these results:

- coefficients, b – column estimate.
- 95% CI – columns conf.low and conf.high.
- p-value – column p.value.

7.5.4   Model fit assessment

It is important to assess to what extend the SLR model reflects the data. First, we can assess this by R^2, which is the percentage of the variance for the outcome that is explained by the predictor. In simpler words, to what extend the variation in the values of the outcome is caused/explained by the predictor. This ranges from 0% (the

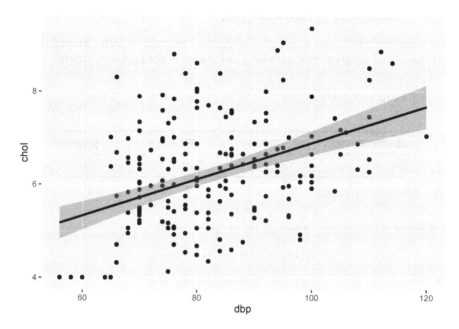

FIGURE 7.2
Scatter plot of `chol` (outcome) vs `dbp` (predictor).

predictor does not explain the outcome at all) to 100% (the predictor explains the outcome perfectly). Here, we obtain the R^2 values,

```
rsq(slr_chol)
```

```
## [1] 0.1798257
```

Next, we can assess the model fit by a scatter plot,

```
plot_slr = ggplot(coronary, aes(x = dbp, y = chol)) +
  geom_point() + geom_smooth(method = lm)
plot_slr
```

This plot allows the assessment of normality, linearity and equal variance assumptions. We expect an elliptical/oval shape (normality) and equal scatter of dots above and below the prediction line (equal variance). These aspects indicate a linear relationship between `chol` and `dbp` (linearity).

7.5.5 Presentation and interpretation

To present the result, we can use `tbl_regression()` to come up with a nice table. We use `slr_chol` of the `glm` output with `tbl_regression()` in the `gtsummary` package.

```
tbl_regression(slr_chol)
```

Characteristic	Beta	95% CI[1]	p-value
dbp	0.04	0.03, 0.05	< 0.001

[1]CI = Confidence Interval

It is also very informative to present the model equation,

$$chol = 3.0 + 0.04 \times dbp$$

where we obtain the intercept value from `summary(slr_chol)`.

Based on the R^2 (which was 0.18), table and model equation, we may interpret the results as follows:

- 1mmHg increase in DBP causes 0.04mmol/L increase in cholesterol level.
- DBP explains 18% of the variance in cholesterol level.

7.6 Multiple Linear Regression

7.6.1 About multiple linear regression

Multiple linear regression (MLR) models *linear* relationship between:

- **outcome**: numerical variable.
- **MORE than one predictors**: numerical and categorical variables.

We may formally represent MLR in form of an equation,

$$numerical\ outcome = intercept$$
$$+ coefficients \times numerical\ predictors$$
$$+ coefficients \times categorical\ predictors$$

or in a shorter form,

$$\hat{y} = b_0 + b_1 x_1 + b_2 x_2 + ... + b_p x_p$$

where we have p predictors.

Whenever the predictor is a categorical variable with more than two levels, we use dummy variable(s). There is no issue with binary categorical variable. For the variable with more than two levels, the number of dummy variables (i.e. once turned into several binary variables) equals number of levels minus one. For example, whenever we have four levels, we will obtain three dummy (binary) variables. As we will see later, `glm` will automatically do this for `factor` variable and provide separate estimates for each dummy variable.

7.6.2 Data exploration

Now, for the MLR we are no longer restricted to one predictor. Let's say, we are interested in knowing the relationship between blood pressure (SBP and DBP), age, BMI, race and render as the predictors and the cholesterol level (outcome). As before, we explore the variables by the descriptive statistics,

```
# numerical
coronary %>% select(-id, -cad, -race, -gender) %>% describe()
```

```
##        vars   n    mean    sd median trimmed   mad   min    max range  skew
## sbp       1 200 130.18 19.81 126.00  128.93 17.79 88.00 187.00 99.00  0.53
## dbp       2 200  82.31 12.90  80.00   81.68 14.83 56.00 120.00 64.00  0.42
## chol      3 200   6.20  1.18   6.19    6.18  1.18  4.00   9.35  5.35  0.18
## age       4 200  47.33  7.34  47.00   47.27  8.15 32.00  62.00 30.00  0.05
## bmi       5 200  37.45  2.68  37.80   37.65  2.37 28.99  45.03 16.03 -0.55
##        kurtosis   se
## sbp       -0.37 1.40
## dbp       -0.33 0.91
## chol      -0.31 0.08
## age       -0.78 0.52
## bmi        0.42 0.19
```

```
# categorical
coronary %>% dplyr::select(race, gender) %>% tbl_summary()
```

Characteristic	N = 200[1]
race	
malay	73 (36%)
chinese	64 (32%)
indian	63 (32%)
gender	
woman	100 (50%)
man	100 (50%)

[1]n (%)

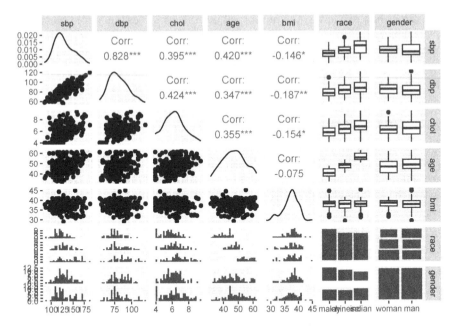

FIGURE 7.3
Pairs plot for all variables.

and the pairs plot, where we focus on the distribution of the data by histograms and box-and-whiskers plots. The pairs plot also includes information on the bivariate correlation statistics between the numerical variables.

```
coronary %>% select(-id, -cad) %>% ggpairs()
```

7.6.3 Univariable analysis

For the univariable analysis in the context of MLR, we aim to select variables that are worthwhile to be included in the multivariable model.

In the context of **exploratory research**, we want to choose only variables with p-values < 0.25 to be included in MLR. To obtain the p-values, you may perform separate SLRs for each of the predictors (on your own). However, obtaining p-value for each predictor is easy by add1() function. Here, we use likelihood ratio test (LRT) using test = "LRT" option to obtain the p-values. We start with an intercept only model slr_chol0 using chol ~ 1 formula specification in the glm followed by add1(). add1() will test each predictor one by one.

```
slr_chol0 = glm(chol ~ 1, data = coronary)  # intercept only model
add1(slr_chol0, scope = ~ sbp + dbp + age + bmi + race + gender,
     test = "LRT")
```

```
## Single term additions
## 
## Model:
## chol ~ 1
##           Df Deviance    AIC scaled dev.  Pr(>Chi)
## <none>        278.77 637.99
## sbp        1  235.36 606.14      33.855 5.938e-09 ***
## dbp        1  228.64 600.34      39.648 3.042e-10 ***
## age        1  243.68 613.08      26.911 2.130e-07 ***
## bmi        1  272.17 635.20       4.792   0.02859 *
## race       2  241.68 613.43      28.561 6.280e-07 ***
## gender     1  277.45 639.04       0.952   0.32933
## ---
## Signif. codes:  0 '***' 0.001 '**' 0.01 '*' 0.05 '.' 0.1 ' ' 1
```

From the output, all variables are important with $p < .25$ except gender. These variables, excluding gender, are candidates in this variable selection step.

However, please keep in mind that in the context of **confirmatory research**, the variables that we want to include are not merely based on p-values alone. It is important to consider expert judgment as well.

7.6.4 Multivariable analysis

Multivariable analysis involves more than one predictors. In the univariable variable selection, we decided on several potential predictors. For MLR, we (judiciously) included these variables in an MLR model. In the present dataset, we have the following considerations:

- including both SBP and DBP is redundant, because both represent the blood pressure. These variables are also highly correlated. This is indicated by the correlation value, $r = 0.828$ and scatter plot for the SBP-DBP pair in the pairs plot in the data exploration step.
- gender was not significant; thus we may exclude the variable.
- let say, as advised by experts in the field, we should exclude age in the modeling.

Now, given these considerations, we perform MLR with the selected variables,

```
mlr_chol = glm(chol ~ dbp + bmi + race, data = coronary)
summary(mlr_chol)
```

```
##
## Call:
## glm(formula = chol ~ dbp + bmi + race, data = coronary)
##
## Deviance Residuals:
##      Min        1Q    Median        3Q       Max
## -2.18698  -0.73076  -0.01935   0.63476   2.91524
##
## Coefficients:
##              Estimate Std. Error t value Pr(>|t|)
## (Intercept)  4.870859   1.245373   3.911 0.000127 ***
## dbp          0.029500   0.006203   4.756 3.83e-06 ***
## bmi         -0.038530   0.028099  -1.371 0.171871
## racechinese  0.356642   0.181757   1.962 0.051164 .
## raceindian   0.724716   0.190625   3.802 0.000192 ***
## ---
## Signif. codes:  0 '***' 0.001 '**' 0.01 '*' 0.05 '.' 0.1 ' ' 1
##
## (Dispersion parameter for gaussian family taken to be 1.083909)
##
##     Null deviance: 278.77  on 199  degrees of freedom
## Residual deviance: 211.36  on 195  degrees of freedom
## AIC: 590.63
##
## Number of Fisher Scoring iterations: 2
```

From the output above, for each variable, we focus these results:

- coefficients, bs – column `estimate`.
- 95% CIs – columns `conf.low` and `conf.high`.
- *p*-values – column `p.value`.

Note that for a categorical variable with more than two categories, the estimates are obtained for each dummy variable. In our case, `race` consists of Malay, Chinese and Indian. From the output, the dummy variables are `racechinese` representing Chinese vs Malay and `raceindian` representing Indian vs Malay dummy variables, where Malay is set as the baseline comparison group.

We also notice that some variables are not significant at significance level of 0.05, namely `bmi` and `racechinese`. As for `racechinese` dummy variable, because this forms part of the `race` variable, we accept the variable because it is marginally insignificant (0.0512 vs 0.05) and the other dummy variable `raceindian` is significant.

Stepwise automatic variable selection

We noted that not all variables included in the model are significant. In our case, we may remove `bmi` because it is not statistically significant. But in exploratory research where we have hundreds of variables, it is impossible to select variables by eye-ball judgment. So, in this case, how to perform the variable selection? To explore the significance of the variables, we may perform stepwise automatic selection. It is important to know stepwise selection is meant for exploratory research. For confirmatory analysis, it is important to rely on expert opinion for the variable selection. We may perform forward, backward or both forward and backward selection combined.

Forward selection starts with an intercept only or empty model without variable. It proceeds by adding one variable after another. In R, Akaike information criterion (AIC) is used as the comparative goodness-of-fit measure and model quality. In the stepwise selection, it seeks to find the model with the lowest AIC iteratively and the steps are shown in the output. More information about AIC can be referred to Hu (2007) and Wikipedia (2022).

```
# forward
mlr_chol_stepforward = step(slr_chol0, scope = ~ dbp + bmi + race,
                            direction = "forward")
```

```
## Start:  AIC=637.99
## chol ~ 1
##
##          Df Deviance    AIC
## + dbp     1   228.64 600.34
## + race    2   241.68 613.43
## + bmi     1   272.17 635.20
## <none>        278.77 637.99
##
## Step:  AIC=600.34
## chol ~ dbp
##
##          Df Deviance    AIC
## + race    2   213.40 590.55
## <none>        228.64 600.34
## + bmi     1   227.04 600.94
##
## Step:  AIC=590.55
## chol ~ dbp + race
##
##          Df Deviance    AIC
## <none>        213.40 590.55
## + bmi     1   211.36 590.63
```

Backward selection starts with a model containing all variables. Then, it proceeds by removing one variable after another, of which it aims to find the model with the lowest AIC.

```
# backward
mlr_chol_stepback = step(mlr_chol, direction = "backward")
```

```
## Start:  AIC=590.63
## chol ~ dbp + bmi + race
##
##           Df Deviance    AIC
## - bmi   1   213.40 590.55
## <none>      211.36 590.63
## - race  2   227.04 600.94
## - dbp   1   235.88 610.58
##
## Step:  AIC=590.55
## chol ~ dbp + race
##
##           Df Deviance    AIC
## <none>      213.40 590.55
## - race  2   228.64 600.34
## - dbp   1   241.68 613.43
```

Bidirectional selection, as implemented in R, starts as with the model with all variables. Then, it proceeds with removing or adding variables, which combines both forward and backward selection methods. It stops once it finds the model with the lowest AIC.

```
# both
mlr_chol_stepboth = step(mlr_chol, direction = "both")
```

```
## Start:  AIC=590.63
## chol ~ dbp + bmi + race
##
##           Df Deviance    AIC
## - bmi   1   213.40 590.55
## <none>      211.36 590.63
## - race  2   227.04 600.94
## - dbp   1   235.88 610.58
##
## Step:  AIC=590.55
## chol ~ dbp + race
##
##           Df Deviance    AIC
## <none>      213.40 590.55
## + bmi   1   211.36 590.63
```

```
## - race   2    228.64 600.34
## - dbp    1    241.68 613.43
```

Preliminary model

Let say, after considering the *p*-value, stepwise selection (in exploratory research) and expert opinion, we decided that our preliminary model is,

```
chol ~ dbp + race
```

and we fit the model again to view basic information of the model,

```
mlr_chol_sel = glm(chol ~ dbp + race, data = coronary)
summary(mlr_chol_sel)
```

```
##
## Call:
## glm(formula = chol ~ dbp + race, data = coronary)
##
## Deviance Residuals:
##     Min       1Q   Median       3Q      Max
## -2.1378  -0.7068  -0.0289   0.5997   2.7778
##
## Coefficients:
##              Estimate Std. Error t value Pr(>|t|)
## (Intercept) 3.298028   0.486213   6.783 1.36e-10 ***
## dbp         0.031108   0.006104   5.096 8.14e-07 ***
## racechinese 0.359964   0.182149   1.976 0.049534 *
## raceindian  0.713690   0.190883   3.739 0.000243 ***
## ---
## Signif. codes:  0 '***' 0.001 '**' 0.01 '*' 0.05 '.' 0.1 ' ' 1
##
## (Dispersion parameter for gaussian family taken to be 1.088777)
##
##     Null deviance: 278.77  on 199  degrees of freedom
## Residual deviance: 213.40  on 196  degrees of freedom
## AIC: 590.55
##
## Number of Fisher Scoring iterations: 2
```

```
rsq(mlr_chol_sel)
```

```
## [1] 0.2345037
```

7.6.5   Interaction

Interaction is the combination of predictors that requires interpretation of their regression coefficients separately based on the levels of the predictor. For example, we need separate interpretation of the coefficient for dbp depending on race group: Malay, Chinese or Indian. This makes interpreting our analysis complicated as we can no longer interpret each coefficient on its own. So, most of the time, we pray not to have interaction in our regression model. We fit the model with a two-way interaction term,

```
summary(glm(chol ~ dbp * race, data = coronary))
```

```
##
## Call:
## glm(formula = chol ~ dbp * race, data = coronary)
##
## Deviance Residuals:
##       Min        1Q    Median        3Q       Max
## -2.10485  -0.77524  -0.02423   0.58059   2.74380
##
## Coefficients:
##                  Estimate Std. Error t value Pr(>|t|)
## (Intercept)       2.11114    0.92803   2.275 0.024008 *
## dbp               0.04650    0.01193   3.897 0.000134 ***
## racechinese       1.95576    1.28477   1.522 0.129572
## raceindian        2.41530    1.25766   1.920 0.056266 .
## dbp:racechinese  -0.02033    0.01596  -1.273 0.204376
## dbp:raceindian   -0.02126    0.01529  -1.391 0.165905
## ---
## Signif. codes:  0 '***' 0.001 '**' 0.01 '*' 0.05 '.' 0.1 ' ' 1
##
## (Dispersion parameter for gaussian family taken to be 1.087348)
##
##     Null deviance: 278.77  on 199  degrees of freedom
## Residual deviance: 210.95  on 194  degrees of freedom
## AIC: 592.23
##
## Number of Fisher Scoring iterations: 2
```

From the output, there is no evidence that suggests the presence of interaction because the included interaction term was insignificant. In R, it is easy to fit interaction by *, e.g. dbp * race will automatically includes all variables involved. This is equal to specifying glm(chol ~ dbp + race + dbp:race, data = coronary), where we can use : to include the interaction.

7.6.6 Model fit assessment

For MLR, we assess the model fit by R^2 and histogram and scatter plots of residuals. Residuals, in simple term, are the discrepancies between the observed values (dots) and the predicted values (by the fit MLR model). So, the lesser the discrepancies, the better is the model fit.

Percentage of variance explained, R^2

First, we obtain the R^2 values. In comparison to the R^2 obtained for the SLR, we include adj = TRUE here to obtain an adjusted R^2. The adjusted R^2 here is the R^2 with penalty for the number of predictors p. This discourages including too many variables, which might be unnecessary.

```
rsq(mlr_chol_sel, adj = TRUE)
```

```
## [1] 0.2227869
```

Histogram and box-and-whiskers plot

Second, we plot a histogram and a box-and-whiskers plot to assess the normality of raw/unstandardized residuals of the MLR model. We expect normally distributed residuals to indicate a good fit of the MLR model. Here, we have a normally distributed residuals.

```
rraw_chol = resid(mlr_chol_sel)
hist(rraw_chol)
```

```
boxplot(rraw_chol)
```

Scatter plots

Third, we plot a standardized residuals (Y-axis) vs standardized predicted values (X-axis) plot. Similar to the one for SLR, this plot allows assessment of normality, linearity and equal variance assumptions. The dots should form elliptical/oval shape (normality) and scattered roughly equal above and below the zero line (equal variance). Both these indicate linearity. Our plot below shows that the assumptions are met.

```
rstd_chol = rstandard(mlr_chol_sel)   # standardized residuals
pstd_chol = scale(predict(mlr_chol_sel))   # standardized predicted values
plot(rstd_chol ~ pstd_chol, xlab = "Std predicted", ylab = "Std residuals")
abline(0, 0)   # normal, linear, equal variance
```

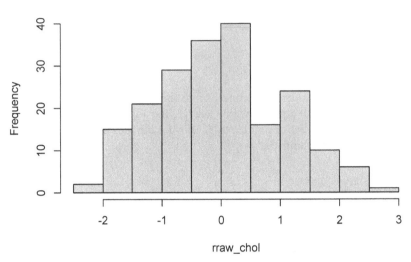

FIGURE 7.4
Histogram of raw residuals.

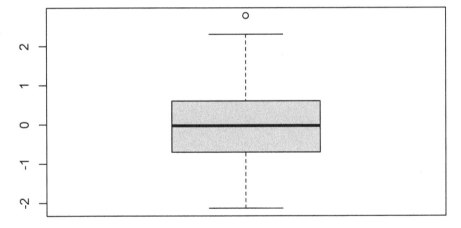

FIGURE 7.5
Box-and-whiskers plot of raw residuals.

In addition to the standardized residuals vs standardized predicted values plot, for numerical predictors, we assess the linear relationship between the raw residuals and the observed values of the numerical predictors. We plot the raw residuals vs numerical predictor below. The plot interpreted in similar way to the standardized

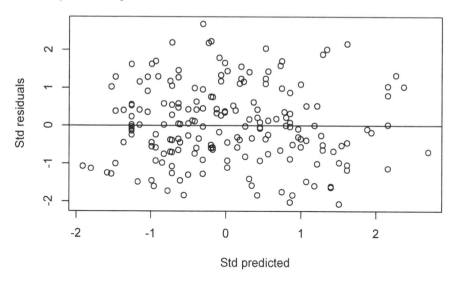

FIGURE 7.6
Scatter plot of standardized residuals vs standardized predicted values.

residuals vs standardized predicted values plot. The plot shows good linearity between the residuals and the numerical predictor.

```
plot(rraw_chol ~ coronary$dbp, xlab = "DBP", ylab = "Raw Residuals")
abline(0, 0)
```

7.6.7 Presentation and interpretation

After passing all the assumption checks, we may now decide on our final model. We may rename the preliminary model `mlr_chol_sel` to `mlr_chol_final` for easier reference.

```
mlr_chol_final = mlr_chol_sel
```

Similar to SLR, we use `tbl_regression()` to come up with a nice table to present the results.

```
tbl_regression(mlr_chol_final)
```

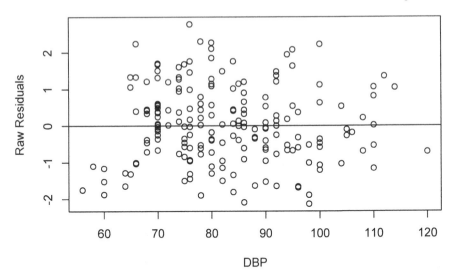

FIGURE 7.7
Scatter plot of raw residuals vs DBP (numerical predictor).

Characteristic	Beta	95% CI[1]	p-value
dbp	0.03	0.02, 0.04	< 0.001
race			
malay	—	—	
chinese	0.36	0.00, 0.72	0.050
indian	0.71	0.34, 1.1	< 0.001

[1]CI = Confidence Interval

It will be useful to be able to save the output in the spreadsheet format for later use.
We can use tidy() function in this case and export it to a .csv file,

```
tib_mlr = tidy(mlr_chol_final, conf.int = TRUE)
write.csv(tib_mlr, "mlr_final.csv")
```

Then, we present the model equation. Cholesterol level in mmol/L can be predicted
by its predictors as given by,

$$chol = 3.30 + 0.03 \times dbp + 0.36 \times race\,(chinese) + 0.71 \times race\,(indian)$$

Based on the adjusted R^2, table and model equation, we may interpret the results as
follows:

- 1mmHg increase in DBP causes 0.03mmol/L increase in cholesterol, while controlling for the effect of race.
- Likewise, 10mmHg increase in DBP causes 0.03 x 10 = 0.3mmol/L increase in cholesterol, while controlling for the effect of race.
- Being Chinese causes 0.36mmol/L increase in cholesterol in comparison to Malay, while controlling for the effect of DBP.
- Being Indian causes 0.71mmol/L increase in cholesterol in comparison to Malay, while controlling for the effect of DBP.
- DBP and race explains 22.3% variance in cholesterol.

For each of this interpretation, please keep in mind to also consider the 95% CI of each of coefficient. For example, being Indian causes 0.71mmol/L increase in cholesterol in comparison to Malay, where this may range from 0.34mmol/L to 1.1mmol/L based on the 95% CI.

7.7 Prediction

In some situations, it is useful to use the SLR/MLR model for prediction. For example, we may want to predict the cholesterol level of a patient given some clinical characteristics. We can use the final model above for prediction. For starter, let us view the predicted values for our sample,

```
coronary$pred_chol = predict(mlr_chol_final)
head(coronary)
```

```
##    id    cad sbp dbp   chol age  bmi   race gender pred_chol
## 1   1 no cad 106  68 6.5725  60 38.9 indian  woman  6.127070
## 2  14 no cad 130  78 6.3250  34 37.8  malay  woman  5.724461
## 3  56 no cad 136  84 5.9675  36 40.5  malay  woman  5.911109
## 4  61 no cad 138 100 7.0400  45 37.6  malay  woman  6.408839
## 5  62 no cad 115  85 6.6550  53 40.3 indian    man  6.655908
## 6  64 no cad 124  72 5.9675  43 37.6  malay    man  5.537812
```

Compare the predicted values with the observed cholesterol level. Recall that we already checked this for the model fit assessment before.

It is more useful to predict for newly observed data. Let us try predicting the cholesterol level for an Indian patient with DBP = 90mmHg,

```
predict(mlr_chol_final, list(dbp = 90, race = "indian"))
```

```
##          1
## 6.811448
```

Now, we also do so the data with many more patients,

```
new_data = data.frame(dbp = c(90, 90, 90),
                      race = c("malay", "chinese", "indian"))
predict(mlr_chol_final, new_data)
```

```
##         1        2        3
## 6.097758 6.457722 6.811448
```

```
new_data$pred_chol = predict(mlr_chol_final, new_data)
new_data
```

```
##    dbp    race pred_chol
## 1   90   malay  6.097758
## 2   90 chinese  6.457722
## 3   90  indian  6.811448
```

7.8   Summary

In this chapter, we went through the basics about SLR and MLR. We performed the analysis for each and learned how to assess the model fit for the regression models. We learned how to nicely present and interpret the results. In addition, we also learned how to utilize the model for prediction. Excellent texts on regression includes Biostatistics: Basic Concepts and Methodology for the Health Sciences (Daniel and Cross, 2014) and the more advanced books such as Applied Linear Statistical Models (Neter et al., 2013) and Epidemiology: Study Design and Data Analysis (Woodward, 2013).

8

Binary Logistic Regression

8.1 Objectives

At the end of the chapter, the readers will be able

- to understand the concept of simple and multiple binary logistic regression
- to perform simple binary logistic regression
- to perform multiple binary logistic regression
- to perform model assessment of binary logistic regression
- to present and interpret results from binary logistic regression

8.2 Introduction

A binary variable is a categorical outcome that has two categories or levels. In medical and health research, the binary outcome variable is very common. Some examples where the outcome is binary include:

- survival status; when the status of cancer patients at the end of treatment is coded as either alive or dead
- relapse status; when the status of a patient is coded as either relapse or not relapse
- satisfaction level; when patients who come to clinics are asked if they are satisfied or not satisfied with the service
- glucose control; when patients were categorized as either good control or poor control based on Hba1c

In statistics, the logistic model (or logit model) is a statistical model that models the probability of an event taking place by having the log-odds for the event be a linear combination of one or more independent variables. In a binary logistic regression model, the dependent variable has two levels (categorical).

8.3   Logistic Regression Model

The logistic model (or logit model) is used to model the probability of a particular class or event existing, such as pass or fail, win or lose, alive or dead or healthy or sick.

More specifically, binary logistic regression is used to model the relationship between a covariate or a set of covariates and an outcome variable which is a binary variable.

8.4   Dataset

We will use a dataset named `stroke.dta` which in STATA format. These data come from a study of hospitalized stroke patients. The original dataset contains 12 variables, but our main variables of interest are:

- status : Status of a patient during hospitalization (alive or dead)
- gcs : Glasgow Coma Scale on admission (range from 3 to 15)
- stroke_type : IS (Ischemic Stroke) or HS (Hemorrhagic Stroke)
- sex : female or male
- dm : History of Diabetes (yes or no)
- sbp : Systolic Blood Pressure (mmHg)
- age : age of patient on admission

The outcome variable is variable status. It is labeled as either dead or alive, which is the outcome of each patient during hospitalization.

8.5   Logit and Logistic Models

The simple binary logit and logistic models refer to a a model with only one covariate (also known as independent variable). For example, if the covariate is gcs (Glasgow Coma Scale), the simple logit model is written as:

$$\hat{g}(x) = ln\left[\frac{\hat{\pi}(x)}{1 - \hat{\pi}(x)}\right]$$

where $\hat{g}(x)$ is the log odds for death for a given value of gcs. And the odds for death for a given value of GCS is written as $= \hat{\beta}_0 + \hat{\beta}_1(gcs)$

And the simple logistic model is also written as:

$$\hat{\pi}(x) = \frac{exp^{\hat{\beta}_0 + \hat{\beta}_1 gcs}}{1 + exp^{\hat{\beta}_0 + \hat{\beta}_1 gcs}}$$

The $\pi(x) = E(Y|x)$ represents the conditional mean of Y given x when the logistic distribution is used. This is also simply known as the predicted probability of death for given value of gcs.

If we have decided (based on our clinical expertise and literature review) that a model that could explain death consists of gcs, stroke type, sex, dm, age and sbp, then the logit model can be expanded to:

$$\hat{g}(x) = \hat{\beta}_0 + \hat{\beta}_1(gcs) + \hat{\beta}_2(stroketype) + \hat{\beta}_3(sex) + \hat{\beta}_4(dm) + \hat{\beta}_5(sbp) + \hat{\beta}_6(age)$$

These are the odds for death given certain gcs, sbp and age values and specific categories of stroke type, sex and diabetes. While the probability of death is

$$\hat{\pi}(x) = \frac{exp^{\hat{\beta}_0 + \hat{\beta}_1(gcs) + \hat{\beta}_2(stroketype) + \hat{\beta}_3(sex) + \hat{\beta}_4(dm) + \hat{\beta}_5(sbp) + \hat{\beta}_6(age)}}{1 + exp^{\hat{\beta}_0 + \hat{\beta}_1(gcs) + \hat{\beta}_2(stroketype) + \hat{\beta}_3(sex) + \hat{\beta}_4(dm) + \hat{\beta}_5(sbp) + \hat{\beta}_6(age)}}$$

In many datasets, some independent variables are either discrete or nominal scale variables. Such variables include race, sex, treatment group, and age categories. Including them in the model is inappropriate as if they were interval scale variables is inappropriate. In some statistical software, these variables are represented by numbers. However, be careful; these numbers are used merely as identifiers or labels for the groups.

In this situation, we will use a method called design variables (or dummy variables). Suppose, for example, assuming that one of the independent variables is obesity type, which is now coded as "Class 1", "Class 2" and "Class 3". In this case, there are 3 levels or categories, hence two design variables $(D - 1)$ are necessary, let's say D1 and D2. One possible coding strategy is that when the patient is in "Class 1" then the two design variables, for D1 and D2 would both be set equal to zero. In this example, "Class 1" is the reference category. When the patient is in "Class 2", then D1 is set as 1 and D2 as 0; when the patient is in "Class 3", then we will set D1 as 0 and D2 and 1. All these coding assignments can be done automatically in the software. But to interpret, we must know which category is the reference.

8.6 Prepare Environment for Analysis

8.6.1 Creating a RStudio project

Start a new analysis task by creating a new RStudio project. To do this,

1. Go to File
2. Click New Project
3. Choose New Directory or Existing Directory.

This directory points to the folder that usually contains the dataset to be analyzed. This is called as the working directory. Make sure there is a folder named as `data` in the folder. If there is not, create one. Make sure the dataset `stroke.dta` is inside the `data` folder in the working directory.

8.6.2   Loading libraries

Next, we will load the necessary packages. We will use 5 packages

1. the built in **stat** package - to run Generalized Linear Model. This is already loaded by default.
2. **haven** - to read SPSS, STATA and SAS dataset
3. **tidyverse** - to perform data transformation
4. **gtsummary** - to provide nice results in a table
5. **broom** - to tidy up the results
6. **LogisticDx** - to do model assessment
7. **here** - to ensure proper directory

To load these packages, we will use the function `library()`:

```
library(haven)
library(tidyverse)
```

```
## -- Attaching core tidyverse packages ----------------------- tidyverse 2.0.0 -
-
## v dplyr      1.1.1      v readr      2.1.4
## v forcats    1.0.0      v stringr    1.5.0
## v ggplot2    3.4.2      v tibble     3.2.1
## v lubridate 1.9.2      v tidyr      1.3.0
## v purrr      1.0.1
##          --        Conflicts       -----------------------------------------
tidyverse_conflicts() --
## x dplyr::filter() masks stats::filter()
## x dplyr::lag()    masks stats::lag()
##     i    Use     the     conflicted     package     (<http://conflicted.r-
lib.org/>) to force all conflicts to become errors
```

```
library(gtsummary)
```

```
## #BlackLivesMatter
```

```
library(broom)
library(LogisticDx)
library(here)
```

```
## here() starts at C:/Users/drkim/Downloads/multivar_data_analysis/multivar_data_analysis
```

8.7   Read Data

WE will read data in the working directory into our R environment. The example dataset comes from a study among stroke inpatients. The dataset is in the STATA format stroke.dta.

```
fatal <- read_dta(here('data','stroke.dta'))
```

Take a peek at data to check for

- variable names
- variable types

```
glimpse(fatal)
```

```
## Rows: 226
## Columns: 7
## $ sex         <dbl+lbl> 1, 1, 1, 2, 1, 2, 2, 1, 2, 2, 1, 2, 2, 2, 2, 1, 2, 1, ~
## $ status      <dbl+lbl> 1, 1, 1, 1, 1, 1, 2, 1, 1, 2, 1, 1, 1, 1, 1, 1, 1, 1, ~
## $ gcs         <dbl> 13, 15, 15, 15, 15, 15, 13, 15, 15, 10, 15, 15, 15, 15, 15~
## $ sbp         <dbl> 143, 150, 152, 215, 162, 169, 178, 180, 186, 185, 122, 211~
## $ dm          <dbl+lbl> 0, 0, 0, 1, 1, 1, 1, 0, 1, 1, 0, 1, 1, 1, 0, 1, 1, 1, ~
## $ age         <dbl> 50, 58, 64, 50, 65, 78, 66, 72, 61, 64, 63, 59, 64, 62, 40~
## $ stroke_type <dbl+lbl> 0, 0, 0, 0, 0, 0, 0, 0, 0, 0, 0, 0, 0, 0, 0, 0, 0, 0, ~
```

8.8   Explore Data

Variables sex, status, dm and stroke type are labeled variables though they are coded as numbers. The numbers represent the groups or categories or levels of the variables. They are categorical variables and not real numbers.

We will transform all of labeled variables to factor variables using `mutate()`. We can quickly achieve that by using the function `across()`. See the codes below to transform all labeled variables in the dataset to factor variables:

```
fatal <-
  fatal %>%
  mutate(across(where(is.labelled), as_factor))
```

Now, examine the summary statistics:

```
fatal %>%
  tbl_summary() %>%
  as_gt()
```

Characteristic	N = 226[1]
sex	
male	97 (43%)
female	129 (57%)
alive or dead	
alive	171 (76%)
dead	55 (24%)
earliest Glasgow Coma Scale	15.0 (10.0, 15.0)
earliest systolic BP (mmHg)	161 (143, 187)
diabetes (yes or no)	138 (61%)
age in years	61 (52, 69)
Ischemic Stroke or Hemorrhagic	
Ischemic Stroke	149 (66%)
Hemorrhagic	77 (34%)

[1]n (%); Median (IQR)

If we want to get summary statistics based on the status of patients at discharge:

```
fatal %>%
  tbl_summary(by = status) %>%
  as_gt()
```

Characteristic	alive, N = 171[1]	dead, N = 55[1]
sex		
male	81 (47%)	16 (29%)
female	90 (53%)	39 (71%)
earliest Glasgow Coma Scale	15.0 (14.0, 15.0)	8.0 (5.0, 11.0)
earliest systolic BP (mmHg)	160 (143, 186)	162 (140, 199)
diabetes (yes or no)	100 (58%)	38 (69%)
age in years	61 (53, 68)	62 (50, 73)
Ischemic Stroke or Hemorrhagic		
Ischemic Stroke	132 (77%)	17 (31%)
Hemorrhagic	39 (23%)	38 (69%)

[1]n (%); Median (IQR)

8.9 Estimate the Regression Parameters

As we assume the outcome variable (status) follows binomial distribution, we will perform binary logistic regression. Logistic regression allow us to estimate the regression parameters $\hat{\beta}_s$ or the log odds in a dataset where the outcome follows binomial or bernoulli distribution.

To achieve the objective above, we do this in two steps:

- The simple binary logistic regression or the univariable logistic regression: In this analysis, there is only one independent variable or covariate in the model. This is also known as the crude or unadjusted analysis.
- The multiple binary logistic regression or the multivariable logistic regression: Here, we expand our model and include two or more independent variables (covariates). The multiple binary logistic regression model is an adjusted model, and we can obtain the estimate of a particular covariate independent of the other covariates in the model.

8.10 Simple Binary Logistic Regression

Simple binary logistic regression model has a dependent variable and only one independent (covariate) variable.

In our dataset, for example, we are interested to model a simple binary logistic regression using

- status as the dependent variable.
- gcs as the independent variable.

The independent variable can be a numerical or a categorical variable.

To estimate the log odds (the regression parameters, β) for the covariate Glasgow Coma Scale (GCS), we can write the logit model as:

$$log\frac{p(status = dead)}{1 - p(status = dead)} = \hat{\beta}_0 + \hat{\beta}_1(gcs)$$

In R, we use the `glm()` function to estimate the regression parameters and other parameters of interest. Let's run the model with gcs as the covariate and name the model as `fatal_glm_1`

```
fatal_glm_1 <-
  glm(status ~ gcs,
      data = fatal,
      family = binomial(link = 'logit'))
```

To get the summarized result of the model `fatal_glm_1`, we will use the `summary()` function:

```
summary(fatal_glm_1)
```

```
##
## Call:
## glm(formula = status ~ gcs, family = binomial(link = "logit"),
##     data = fatal)
##
## Deviance Residuals:
##     Min      1Q   Median      3Q     Max
## -2.1179  -0.3921  -0.3921  -0.3921  2.2820
##
## Coefficients:
##             Estimate Std. Error z value Pr(>|z|)
## (Intercept)  3.29479    0.60432   5.452 4.98e-08 ***
## gcs         -0.38811    0.05213  -7.446 9.64e-14 ***
## ---
## Signif. codes:  0 '***' 0.001 '**' 0.01 '*' 0.05 '.' 0.1 ' ' 1
##
## (Dispersion parameter for binomial family taken to be 1)
##
##     Null deviance: 250.83  on 225  degrees of freedom
## Residual deviance: 170.92  on 224  degrees of freedom
```

```
## AIC: 174.92
##
## Number of Fisher Scoring iterations: 5
```

To get the model summary in a data frame format, so we can edit more easily, we can use the `tidy()` function from the **broom** package. The package also contains other functions to provide other parameters useful for us later.

The function `conf.int()` will provide the confidence intervals (CI). The default is set at the 95 level:

```
tidy(fatal_glm_1, conf.int = TRUE)
```

```
## # A tibble: 2 x 7
##   term        estimate std.error statistic  p.value conf.low conf.high
##   <chr>          <dbl>     <dbl>     <dbl>    <dbl>    <dbl>     <dbl>
## 1 (Intercept)    3.29     0.604      5.45 4.98e- 8     2.17      4.55
## 2 gcs           -0.388    0.0521    -7.45 9.64e-14    -0.497    -0.292
```

The estimates here are the log odds for death for a given value of gcs. In this example, each unit increase in gcs, the crude or unadjusted log odds for death due to stroke change by a factor -0.388 with 95 CI ranges from $-0.497 and -0.292$.

Now, let's use another covariate, `stroke_type`. Stroke type has 2 levels or categories; Hemorrhagic Stroke (HS) and Ischemic Stroke (IS). HS is known to cause a higher risk for deaths in stroke. We will model stroke type (`stroke_type`), name the model as `fatal_glm_2` and show the result using `tidy()`

```
fatal_glm_2 <-
  glm(status ~ stroke_type,
      data = fatal,
      family = binomial(link = 'logit'))
tidy(fatal_glm_2, conf.int = TRUE)
```

```
## # A tibble: 2 x 7
##   term                estimate std.error statistic  p.value conf.low conf.high
##   <chr>                  <dbl>     <dbl>     <dbl>    <dbl>    <dbl>     <dbl>
## 1 (Intercept)           -2.05     0.258     -7.95 1.80e-15    -2.59     -1.57
## 2 stroke_typeHaemorrha~  2.02     0.344      5.88 4.05e- 9     1.36      2.72
```

The simple binary logistic regression model show that patients with Hemorrhagic Stroke (HS) had a higher log odds for death during admission (by a factor 2.02) as compared to patients with Ischemic Stroke (IS).

8.11   Multiple Binary Logistic Regression

There are multiple factors that can contribute to the outcomes of stroke. Hence, there is a strong motivation to include other independent variables or covariates to the model. For example, in the case of stroke:

- It is unlikely that only one variable (gcs or stroke type) is related to stroke. Stroke like other cardiovascular diseases has many factors affecting the outcome. It makes more sense to consider adding other independent variables that we believe are important independent variables for stroke outcome in the model.
- by adding more covariates in the model, we can estimate the adjusted log odds. These log odds indicate the relationship of a particular covariate independent of other covariates in the model. In epidemiology, we always can this as adjustment. An adjustment is important particularly when we have confounding effects from other independent variables.
- interaction term can be generated (the product of two covariates) and added to the model to be estimated.

To add or not to add variables is a big subject on its own. Usually it is governed by clinical experience, subject matter experts and some preliminary analysis. You may read the last chapter of the book to understand more about model building and variable selection.

Let's expand our model and include gcs, stroke type, sex, dm, sbp and age in the model. We will name this model as `fatal_mv`. As we have more than one independent variables in the model, we will call this as multiple binary logistic regression.

To estimates the multiple logistic regression model in R:

```
fatal_mv1 <-
  glm(status ~ gcs + stroke_type + sex + dm + sbp + age,
      data = fatal,
      family = binomial(link = 'logit'))
summary(fatal_mv1)


##
## Call:
## glm(formula = status ~ gcs + stroke_type + sex + dm + sbp + age,
##     family = binomial(link = "logit"), data = fatal)
##
## Deviance Residuals:
##     Min       1Q   Median       3Q      Max
## -2.3715  -0.4687  -0.3280  -0.1921   2.5150
##
```

```
## Coefficients:
##                            Estimate Std. Error z value Pr(>|z|)
## (Intercept)              -0.1588269  1.6174965  -0.098  0.92178
## gcs                      -0.3284640  0.0557574  -5.891 3.84e-09 ***
## stroke_typeHaemorrhagic   1.2662764  0.4365882   2.900  0.00373 **
## sexfemale                 0.4302901  0.4362742   0.986  0.32399
## dmyes                     0.4736670  0.4362309   1.086  0.27756
## sbp                       0.0008612  0.0060619   0.142  0.88703
## age                       0.0242321  0.0154010   1.573  0.11562
## ---
## Signif. codes:  0 '***' 0.001 '**' 0.01 '*' 0.05 '.' 0.1 ' ' 1
##
## (Dispersion parameter for binomial family taken to be 1)
##
##     Null deviance: 250.83  on 225  degrees of freedom
## Residual deviance: 159.34  on 219  degrees of freedom
## AIC: 173.34
##
## Number of Fisher Scoring iterations: 5
```

We could get a cleaner result in a data frame format (and you can edit in spreadsheet easily) of the multivariable model by using `tidy()` function:

```
log_odds <- tidy(fatal_mv1,
                 conf.int = TRUE)
log_odds
```

```
## # A tibble: 7 x 7
##   term              estimate std.error statistic p.value conf.low conf.high
##   <chr>                <dbl>     <dbl>     <dbl>   <dbl>    <dbl>     <dbl>
## 1 (Intercept)       -1.59e-1     1.62   -0.0982 9.22e-1   -3.38      3.01
## 2 gcs               -3.28e-1     0.0558  -5.89  3.84e-9   -0.444    -0.224
## 3 stroke_typeHaemorrhag~ 1.27e+0  0.437   2.90  3.73e-3    0.411     2.13
## 4 sexfemale          4.30e-1     0.436    0.986 3.24e-1   -0.420     1.30
## 5 dmyes              4.74e-1     0.436    1.09  2.78e-1   -0.368     1.35
## 6 sbp                8.61e-4     0.00606  0.142 8.87e-1   -0.0110    0.0129
## 7 age                2.42e-2     0.0154   1.57  1.16e-1   -0.00520   0.0555
```

We could see that the multivariable model that we named as `fatal_mv1`, can be interpreted as below:

- with one unit increase in Glasgow Coma Scale (GCS), the log odds for death during hospitalization equals to −0.328, adjusting for other covariates.
- patients with HS have 1.266 times the log odds for death as compared to patients with IS, adjusting for other covariates.

- female patients have 0.430 times the log odds for death as compared to male patients, adjusting for other covariates.
- patients with diabetes mellitus have 0.474 times the log odds for deaths as compared to patients with no diabetes mellitus.
- With one mmHg increase in systolic blood pressure, the log odds for deaths change by a factor of 0.00086, when adjusting for other variables.

- with an increase in one year of age, the log odds for deaths change by a factor of 0.024, when adjusting for other variables.

In this book, we use the term independent variables, covariates and predictors interchangeably.

8.12   Convert the Log Odds to Odds Ratio

Lay person has difficulty to interpret log odds from logistic regression. That's why, it is more common to interpret the logistic regression models using odds ratio. To obtain the odds ratios, we set the argument exponentiate = TRUE in the tidy() function. Actually, odds ratio can be easily calculate by $\exp^{\beta_i}$

```
odds_ratio <- tidy(fatal_mv1,
                   exponentiate = TRUE,
                   conf.int = TRUE)
odds_ratio
```

```
## # A tibble: 7 x 7
##   term               estimate std.error statistic p.value conf.low conf.high
##   <chr>                 <dbl>     <dbl>     <dbl>   <dbl>    <dbl>     <dbl>
## 1 (Intercept)           0.853     1.62    -0.0982 9.22e-1   0.0341      20.3
## 2 gcs                   0.720    0.0558    -5.89  3.84e-9    0.641     0.799
## 3 stroke_typeHaemorrhag~ 3.55    0.437      2.90  3.73e-3    1.51      8.45
## 4 sexfemale             1.54     0.436      0.986 3.24e-1    0.657     3.69
## 5 dmyes                 1.61     0.436      1.09  2.78e-1    0.692     3.87
## 6 sbp                   1.00     0.00606    0.142 8.87e-1    0.989     1.01
## 7 age                   1.02     0.0154     1.57  1.16e-1    0.995     1.06
```

8.13   Making Inference

Let us rename the table appropriately so we can combine the results from the log odds and the odds ratio later.

```
tab_logistic <- bind_cols(log_odds, odds_ratio)
```

```
## New names:
## * `term` -> `term...1`
## * `estimate` -> `estimate...2`
## * `std.error` -> `std.error...3`
## * `statistic` -> `statistic...4`
## * `p.value` -> `p.value...5`
## * `conf.low` -> `conf.low...6`
## * `conf.high` -> `conf.high...7`
## * `term` -> `term...8`
## * `estimate` -> `estimate...9`
## * `std.error` -> `std.error...10`
## * `statistic` -> `statistic...11`
## * `p.value` -> `p.value...12`
## * `conf.low` -> `conf.low...13`
## * `conf.high` -> `conf.high...14`
```

```
tab_logistic %>%
  select(term...1, estimate...2, std.error...3,
         estimate...9, conf.low...13, conf.high...14 ,p.value...5) %>%
  rename(covariate = term...1,
         log_odds = estimate...2,
         SE = std.error...3,
         odds_ratio = estimate...9,
         lower_OR = conf.low...13,
         upper_OR = conf.high...14,
         p.val = p.value...5)
```

```
## # A tibble: 7 x 7
##   covariate                  log_odds       SE odds_ratio lower_OR upper_OR    p.val
##   <chr>                         <dbl>    <dbl>      <dbl>    <dbl>    <dbl>    <dbl>
## 1 (Intercept)                  -0.159   1.62        0.853   0.0341    20.3  9.22e-1
## 2 gcs                          -0.328   0.0558      0.720   0.641     0.799 3.84e-9
## 3 stroke_typeHaemorrhagic       1.27    0.437       3.55    1.51      8.45  3.73e-3
## 4 sexfemale                     0.430   0.436       1.54    0.657     3.69  3.24e-1
## 5 dmyes                         0.474   0.436       1.61    0.692     3.87  2.78e-1
## 6 sbp                           0.000861 0.00606    1.00    0.989     1.01  8.87e-1
## 7 age                          0.0242   0.0154      1.02    0.995     1.06  1.16e-1
```

In the model, we can interpret the estimates as below:

- if **gcs** increases by 1 unit (when *stroke type* is adjusted), the log odds for death changes by a factor -0.32 or the odds for death changes by a factor 0.72 (odds for

death reduces for 28%). The $95\%CI$ are between $21\%, 36\%$, adjusting for other covariates.
- patients with HS have 3.55% times higher odds for stroke deaths - with $95\%CI$: $17\%, 85\%$ - as compared to patients with HS, adjusting for other independent variables.
- female patients have 53% higher odds for death as compared to female patients ($p = 0.154$), adjusting for other covariates.
- patients with diabetes mellitus have 60.6% higher odds for deaths compared to patients with no diabetes mellitus though the p value is above 5% ($p = 0.642\%$).
- With one mmHg increase in systolic blood pressure, the odds for death change by a factor 1.00086, when adjusting for other variables. The p value is also larger than 5%.

- with an increase in one year of age, the odds for deaths increase by a factor of 1.025, when adjusting for other variables. However, the p value is 0.115

8.14   Models Comparison

The importance of independent variables in the models should not be based on their p-values or the Wald statistics alone. It is recommended to use likelihood ratio to compare models. The difference in the likelihood ratio between models can guide us on choosing a better model.

For example, when we compare model 1 (fatal_mv) and model 2 (fatal_glm_1), could we say that they are different? One approach is to see if both models are different statistically. This comparison can be done by setting the level of significance at 5%.

```
anova( fatal_glm_1, fatal_mv1, test = 'Chisq')
```

```
## Analysis of Deviance Table
##
## Model 1: status ~ gcs
## Model 2: status ~ gcs + stroke_type + sex + dm + sbp + age
##    Resid. Df Resid. Dev Df Deviance Pr(>Chi)
## 1        224     170.92
## 2        219     159.34  5   11.582  0.04098 *
## ---
## Signif. codes:  0 '***' 0.001 '**' 0.01 '*' 0.05 '.' 0.1 ' ' 1
```

Both models are different statistically (at 5% level). Hence, we prefer to keep model fatal_mv1 because the model makes more sense (more parsimonious).

Now, let's be economical, and just keep variables such as gcs, stroke type and age in the model. We will name this multivariable logistic model as `fatal_mv2`:

```
fatal_mv2 <-
  glm(status ~ gcs + stroke_type + age,
      data = fatal,
      family = binomial(link = 'logit'))
```

And we will perform model comparison again:

```
anova( fatal_mv1,
       fatal_mv2, test = 'Chisq')


## Analysis of Deviance Table
##
## Model 1: status ~ gcs + stroke_type + sex + dm + sbp + age
## Model 2: status ~ gcs + stroke_type + age
##   Resid. Df Resid. Dev Df Deviance Pr(>Chi)
## 1       219     159.34
## 2       222     161.51 -3  -2.1743   0.537
```

The p-value is above the threshold of 5% set by us. Hence, we do not want to reject the null hypothesis (null hypothesis says that both models are not statistically different). Our approach also agrees with Occam's razor principle; always choose simpler model. In this case, `fatal_mv2` is simpler and deserves further exploration.

8.15 Adding an Interaction Term

Interaction effect occurs when the effect of one variable depends on the value of another variable (in the case of two interacting variables). Interaction effect is common in regression analysis, ANOVA, and in designed experiments.

Two-way interaction term involves two risk factors and their effect on one disease outcome. If the effect of one risk factor is the same within strata defined by the other, then there is no interaction. When the effect of one risk factor is different within strata defined by the other, then there is an interaction; this can be considered as a biological interaction.

Statistical interaction in the regression model can be measured based on the ways that risks are calculated (modeling). The presence of statistical interaction may not reflect true biological interaction.

Let's add an interaction term between stroke type and diabetes:

```
fatal_mv2_ia <-
  glm(status ~ gcs + stroke_type + stroke_type:gcs + age,
      data = fatal,
      family = binomial(link = 'logit'))
tidy(fatal_mv2_ia)
```

```
## # A tibble: 5 x 5
##    term                          estimate std.error statistic  p.value
##    <chr>                            <dbl>     <dbl>     <dbl>    <dbl>
## 1 (Intercept)                      0.508      1.37     0.371    0.710
## 2 gcs                             -0.320     0.0800    -4.01  0.0000619
## 3 stroke_typeHaemorrhagic          1.61       1.30     1.24     0.217
## 4 age                             0.0236    0.0147     1.60     0.109
## 5 gcs:stroke_typeHaemorrhagic     -0.0347    0.111    -0.312    0.755
```

$$\hat{g}(x) = \hat{\beta}_0 + \hat{\beta}_1(gcs) + \hat{\beta}_2(stroketype) + \hat{\beta}_3(age) + \hat{\beta}_4(gcs \times stroke_type)$$

To decide if we should keep an interaction term in the model, we should consider if the interaction term indicates both biological and statistical significance. If we believe that the interaction reflects both, then we should keep the interaction term in the model.

Using our data, we can see that:

- the coefficient for the interaction term for stroke type and gcs is not significant at the level of significance of 5% that we set.
- stroke experts also believe that the effect of gcs on stroke death is not largely different between different stroke type

Using both reasons, we decide not to keep the two-way interaction between gcs and stroke type in our multivariable logistic model.

8.16 Prediction from Binary Logistic Regression

The **broom** package has a function called `augment()` which can calculate:

1. estimated log odds
2. probabilities
3. residuals
4. hat values

5. Cooks distance
6. standardized residuals

8.16.1 Predict the log odds

To obtain the `.fitted` column for the estimated log odds for death of each patient in the stroke data, we can run:

```
log_odds_mv2 <- augment(fatal_mv2)
log_odds_mv2 %>%
  slice(1:10)
```

```
## # A tibble: 10 x 10
##    status   gcs stroke_type      age .fitted .resid    .hat .sigma   .cooksd
##    <fct> <dbl> <fct>          <dbl>   <dbl>  <dbl>   <dbl>  <dbl>     <dbl>
##  1 alive    13 Ischaemic Stroke  50   -2.49 -0.398 0.00991  0.854 0.000209
##  2 alive    15 Ischaemic Stroke  58   -2.98 -0.314 0.00584  0.855 0.0000748
##  3 alive    15 Ischaemic Stroke  64   -2.84 -0.337 0.00590  0.855 0.0000871
##  4 alive    15 Ischaemic Stroke  50   -3.17 -0.287 0.00657  0.855 0.0000698
##  5 alive    15 Ischaemic Stroke  65   -2.82 -0.341 0.00599  0.855 0.0000904
##  6 alive    15 Ischaemic Stroke  78   -2.51 -0.395 0.00980  0.854 0.000203
##  7 dead     13 Ischaemic Stroke  66   -2.12  2.11  0.00831  0.843 0.0176
##  8 alive    15 Ischaemic Stroke  72   -2.65 -0.369 0.00731  0.855 0.000131
##  9 alive    15 Ischaemic Stroke  61   -2.91 -0.325 0.00579  0.855 0.0000796
## 10 dead     10 Ischaemic Stroke  64   -1.15  1.69  0.0173   0.847 0.0141
## # i 1 more variable: .std.resid <dbl>
```

The `slice()` gives the snapshot of the data. In this case, we choose the first 10 patients.

8.16.2 Predict the probabilities

To obtain the `.fitted` column for the estimated probabilities for death of each patient, we specify `type.predict = "response"`:

```
prob_mv2 <-
  augment(fatal_mv2,
          type.predict = "response")
prob_mv2 %>%
  slice(1:10)
```

```
## # A tibble: 10 x 10
##    status   gcs stroke_type      age .fitted .resid    .hat .sigma   .cooksd
##    <fct> <dbl> <fct>          <dbl>   <dbl>  <dbl>   <dbl>  <dbl>     <dbl>
```

```
##  1 alive     13 Ischaemic Stroke    50  0.0763 -0.398 0.00991   0.854 0.000209
##  2 alive     15 Ischaemic Stroke    58  0.0482 -0.314 0.00584   0.855 0.0000748
##  3 alive     15 Ischaemic Stroke    64  0.0551 -0.337 0.00590   0.855 0.0000871
##  4 alive     15 Ischaemic Stroke    50  0.0403 -0.287 0.00657   0.855 0.0000698
##  5 alive     15 Ischaemic Stroke    65  0.0564 -0.341 0.00599   0.855 0.0000904
##  6 alive     15 Ischaemic Stroke    78  0.0750 -0.395 0.00980   0.854 0.000203
##  7 dead      13 Ischaemic Stroke    66  0.107   2.11  0.00831   0.843 0.0176
##  8 alive     15 Ischaemic Stroke    72  0.0658 -0.369 0.00731   0.855 0.000131
##  9 alive     15 Ischaemic Stroke    61  0.0516 -0.325 0.00579   0.855 0.0000796
## 10 dead      10 Ischaemic Stroke    64  0.241   1.69  0.0173    0.847 0.0141
## # i 1 more variable: .std.resid <dbl>
```

8.17   Model Fitness

The basic logistic regression model assessment includes the measurement of overall model fitness. To do this, we check

- area under the curve
- Hosmer-Lemeshow test
- modified Hosmer-Lemeshow test
- Oseo Rojek test

A fit model will not produce a large difference between the observed (from data) and the predicted values (from model). The difference is usually compared using p-values. If the p-values from the fit test show value of bigger than 0.05, then the test indicates that there is no significant difference between the observed data and the predicted values. Hence, it will support that the model has good fit.

```
fit_m <- gof(fatal_mv2,
             g = 8)


## Setting levels: control = 0, case = 1

## Setting direction: controls < cases
```

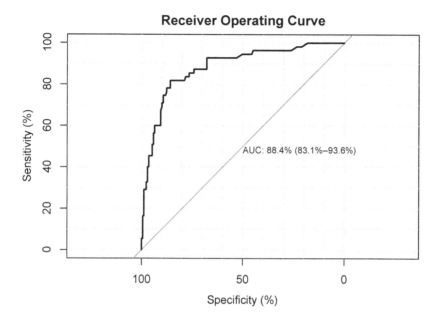

```
fit_m$gof
```

```
##              test  stat      val df       pVal
## 1:             HL chiSq  4.622183  6 0.5930997
## 2:            mHL     F  1.071882  7 0.3844230
## 3:           OsRo     Z -0.501724 NA 0.6158617
## 4: SstPgeq0.5        Z  1.348843 NA 0.1773873
## 5:       SstPl0.5    Z  1.516578 NA 0.1293733
## 6:        SstBoth chiSq  4.119387  2 0.1274931
## 7: SllPgeq0.5 chiSq  1.579811  1 0.2087879
## 8:      SllPl0.5 chiSq  2.311910  1 0.1283862
## 9:       SllBoth chiSq  2.341198  2 0.3101811
```

Our model shows that:

- the area under the curve is 87.2%. The values of above 80 are considered to have good discriminating effect.
- the p-values from the Hosmer Lemeshow, the modified Hosmer Lemeshow and the Oseo Rojek are all above 5% values. This support our believe that our model has good fit.

8.18 Presentation of Logistic Regression Model

The **gtsummary** package has a useful function `tbld_regression()` which can be used to produce a formatted table suitable for publication. For example, to generate a table for adjusted log odds ratio derived from our multivariable logistic regression model `fatal_mv2`, we can use the codes below:

```
tbl_regression(fatal_mv2) %>%
  as_gt()
```

Characteristic	log(OR)[1]	95% CI[1]	p-value
earliest Glasgow Coma Scale	−0.34	−0.45, −0.24	< 0.001
Ischemic Stroke or Hemorrhagic			
Ischemic Stroke	—	—	
Hemorrhagic	1.2	0.38, 2.1	0.004
age in years	0.02	0.00, 0.05	0.11

[1]OR = Odds Ratio, CI = Confidence Interval

Next, to generate the adjusted odds ratios table:

```
tbl_regression(fatal_mv2, exponentiate = TRUE) %>%
  as_gt()
```

Characteristic	OR[1]	95% CI[1]	p-value
earliest Glasgow Coma Scale	0.71	0.64, 0.79	< 0.001
Ischemic Stroke or Hemorrhagic			
Ischemic Stroke	—	—	
Hemorrhagic	3.40	1.46, 7.97	0.004
age in years	1.02	1.00, 1.05	0.11

[1]OR = Odds Ratio, CI = Confidence Interval

8.19 Summary

In this chapter, we briefly explain that when readers want to model the relationship of a single or multiple independent variables with a binary outcome, then one of the analyses of choice is binary logit or logistic regression model. Then, we demonstrated simple and multiple binary logistic regression using `glm()` function and making predictions from the logistic regression model. Lastly, using **gtsummary** package readers can quickly create a nice regression table.

There are a number of good references to help readers understand binary logistic regression better. The references that we list below also contains workflow that will be useful for readers when modeling logistic regression. We highly recommend readers to read Applied Logistic Regression (Hosmer et al., 2013), Logistic Regression: Self Learning Text (Kleinbaum, 2010) to strengthen your theory and concepts on logistic regression. And next you can refer to A Handbook of Statistical Analyses Using R (Everitt and Hothorn, 2017) which provides in greater details the R codes relevant to logistic regression models.

9

Multinomial Logistic Regression

9.1 Objectives

At the end of this chapter, readers should be able:

- to understand the concept of logistic regression model to analyze data with polychotomous (multinomial) outcome
- to estimate parameters of interest in a logistic regression model from data with polychotomous (multinomial) outcome
- to make inference based on a logistic regression model from data with polychotomous (multinomial) outcome
- to predict the outcome based on a logistic regression model from data with polychotomous (multinomial) outcome
- to perform model checking of logistic regression model from data with polychotomous (multinomial) outcomes

9.2 Introduction

Some data come with multinomial outcomes, in which the outcome variable is a nominal or polychotomous variable with more than two levels. In multinomial outcome data, the outcome has no natural ordering. If it has, then it is best treated as an ordinal outcome data. For these data, we can modify the binary logistic model to make estimation and inference (Kleinbaum, 2010; Hosmer et al., 2013).

Variables with more than two levels are known as either:

1. multinomial data
2. polychotomous data
3. polytomous data

If we employ logistic regression to such data, then the analysis is known as polytomous or multinomial logistic regression. Again, the polychotomous outcome does not have any natural order. When the categories of the outcome variable do have a natural order, ordinal logistic regression is preferred.

9.3   Examples of Multinomial Outcome Variables

Examples of data with polychotomous outcome variables (with more than two levels) include:

- disease symptoms that have been classified by subjects as being absent, mild, moderate, or severe,
- tumour invasiveness classified as in situ, locally invasive, ormetastatic, or
- patient preferred treatment regimen, selected from among three or more options for example oral medication only, oral medication plus injection medication or injection only.

A numerical outcome can be categorized based on different cut-off points. The newly created categorical variable is now either treated as a nominal, polychotomous or multinomial outcome, or as an ordinal outcome. That justifies the use of multinomial logistic regression.

9.4   Models for Multinomial Outcome Data

With a multinomial outcome data, an extension of logistic regression know as multinomial logit or multinomial logistic regression can be performed. In multinomial logistic regression, one of the categories of the outcome variable is designated as the reference category and each of the other levels is compared with this reference. The choice of reference category can be arbitrary and is at the discretion of the researcher. Most software set the first category as the reference (also known as the baseline category) by default.

Other models that can analyze data with polychotomous outcome include:

1. Stereotype logistic regression - each independent variable has one value for each individual
2. Alternative-specific variables

9.5 Estimation for Multinomial Logit Model

Remember, interpreting and assessing the significance of the estimated coefficients are the main objectives of regression analysis. in multinomial logistic regression, we would like to model the relationship between covariates with the outcome variable that has more than two categories but without ordering or ranking.

The actual values taken by the dependent variable are irrelevant. In Stata, the **exponentiated beta** $\exp^{\beta}$ will generate the so-called the **relative-risk ratio**. The dependent variable again, is a discrete variable and the model is estimated using maximum likelihood.

In multinomial logistic regression for example in data with three categories of the outcome, the sum of the probabilities for the three outcome categories must be equal to 1 (the total probability). The comparison is done between two categories each time. Because of that, each comparison considers only two probabilities, and the probabilities in the ratio do not sum to 1. Thus, the two odds-like expressions in multinomial logistic regression are not true odds.

Multinomial logistic regression can be thought of as simulteneously fitting binary logits for all comparisons among the alternatives.

9.5.1 Log odds and odds ratios

In the special case where the covariate is binary, coded 0 or 1, we simplify the notation to $OR_j = OR_j(1,0)$. Let's use an example where data have three categories of outcome; 0,1 and 2.

Let's say we have a dataset with the outcome variable, Y, and is coded as 0, 1, or 2. In practice one should check that the software package that is going to be used allows a 0 code as the smallest category. We have used packages that require that the codes begin with 1.

SO the logit functions (log odds) when the outcome is a D variable with (0,1 and 2 values) are as below

1. the log odds for comparison between 0 and 1 is

$$g_1(x) = ln\frac{P(D = 1|X_1)}{P(D = 0|X_1)} = \alpha_1 + (\beta_{11}X_1)$$

2. and, the log odds for comparison between 0 and 2 is

$$g_2(x) = ln\frac{P(D = 2|X_1)}{P(D = 0|X_1)} = \alpha_2 + (\beta_{21}X_1)$$

If for example, we assume that the outcome labeled with $Y = 0$ is the reference outcome. The subscript on the odds ratio indicates which outcome is being compared to the reference category outcome. The odds ratio of outcome $Y = j$ versus $Y = 0$ for the covariate values of $x = a$ versus $x = b$ is:

$$OR_j(a,b) = \frac{Pr(Y = j|x = a)/(Pr(Y = 0|x = a)}{Pr(Y = j|x = b)/Pr(Y = 0|x = b)}$$

Each odds ratio is calculated in a manner similar to that used in standard logistic regression. That is:

$$OR_1(X = 1, X = 0) = \frac{Pr(D = 1|X = 1)/(Pr(D = 0|X = 1)}{Pr(Y = 1|X = 0)/Pr(D = 0|X = 0)} = \exp^{\beta_{11}}$$

$$OR_2(X = 2, X = 0) = \frac{Pr(D = 2|X = 1)/(Pr(D = 0|X = 1)}{Pr(D = 2|X = 0)/Pr(D = 0|X = 0)} = \exp^{\beta_{21}}$$

9.5.2 Conditional probabilities

The conditional probabilities for the multinomial logit model are:

$$Pr(D = 0|x) = \frac{1}{1 + e^{g_1(x)} + e^{g_2(x)}}$$

$$Pr(D = 1|x) = \frac{e^{g_1(x)}}{1 + e^{g_1(x)} + e^{g_2(x)}}$$

$$Pr(D = 2|x) = \frac{e^{g_2(x)}}{1 + e^{g_1(x)} + e^{g_2(x)}}$$

9.6 Prepare Environment

Start brand new analysis with a new project in RStudio. To do so,

- Go to RStudio Menu
- Click File
- Click New Project
- Choose either New Directory or Existing Directory (to point to existing folder usually with the dataset)

9.6.1 Load libraries

We will load

- **here** package that enables easy file referencing
- **tidyverse** for data wrangling and plotting
- **haven** to read data in various statistical formats
- **gtsummary** to produce statistical tables
- **VGAM** package where we will be using the `vglm()` function to perform multinomial logistic regression
- **kableExtra** to produce nice tables for the results

```
library(here)
```

```
## here() starts at C:/Users/drkim/Downloads/multivar_data_analysis/multivar_data_analysis
```

```
library(tidyverse)
```

```
## -- Attaching core tidyverse packages ----------------------- tidyverse 2.0.0 --
## v dplyr      1.1.1      v readr      2.1.4
## v forcats    1.0.0      v stringr    1.5.0
## v ggplot2    3.4.2      v tibble     3.2.1
## v lubridate 1.9.2       v tidyr      1.3.0
## v purrr      1.0.1
## --           Conflicts    ------------------------------------------
tidyverse_conflicts() --
## x dplyr::filter() masks stats::filter()
## x dplyr::lag()    masks stats::lag()
## i   Use    the    conflicted   package    (<http://conflicted.r-
lib.org/>) to force all conflicts to become errors
```

```
library(haven)
library(gtsummary)
library(VGAM)
```

```
## Loading required package: stats4
## Loading required package: splines
```

```
library(kableExtra)
```

```
##
## Attaching package: 'kableExtra'
##
## The following object is masked from 'package:dplyr':
```

```
##
##      group_rows
```

9.6.2 Dataset

The dataset contain all variables of our interest. For the purpose of this assignment, we want to explore the association of hypertension status, weight and total cholesterol with the result of screening FBS. The variables in the datasets as follow:

1. fbs : Fasting Blood Sugar (mmol/L). The data ranges from 2.51 mmol/L to 28.01 mmol/L.
2. totchol : Total Cholesterol (mmol/L). The data ranges from 0.18 mmol/L to 23.14 mmol/L.
3. hpt : Hypertension Status. Coded as Yes and No.
4. weight : Body weight measures in kilogram. The data ranges between 30kg to 187.8kg.

9.6.3 Read data

We will use `haven::read_dta()` function to read stata `.dta` data into the memory. Remember, we can also use `foreign::read.dta()` function to read stata `.dta` data. It is your choice.

We use `here()` to indicate that the folder `data` contains the dataset. And then we specify `metabolic_syndrome.dta` as the dataset to be read.

```
ms <- read_dta(here('data','metabolic_syndrome.dta'))
```

We can then quickly glance at the number of observations and the type of variables in the `ms` dataset.

```
glimpse(ms)
```

```
## Rows: 4,340
## Columns: 21
## $ codesub  <chr> "R-S615112", "MAA615089", "M-M616372", "MFM615361", "R-A61578~
## $ age      <dbl> 70, 20, 29, 25, 37, 43, 26, 28, 48, 20, 56, 55, 26, 39, 18, 2~
## $ hpt      <chr> "yes", "no", "no", "no", "no", "no", "no", "no", "no", "no", ~
## $ smoking  <chr> "never smoked", "still smoking", "never smoked", "still smoki~
## $ dmdx     <chr> "no", "no", "no", "no", "no", "no", "no", "no", "no", "no", "~
## $ height   <dbl> 1.54, 1.74, 1.54, 1.60, 1.44, 1.46, 1.47, 1.61, 1.68, 1.55, 1~
## $ weight   <dbl> 40.0, 54.6, 37.0, 48.4, 44.5, 45.5, 48.0, 40.0, 48.4, 41.0, 5~
## $ waist    <dbl> 76.0, 83.0, 83.0, 83.5, 85.0, 90.0, 91.0, 80.0, 82.0, 79.0, 9~
## $ hip      <dbl> 61, 62, 63, 64, 64, 64, 64, 64, 65, 66, 67, 67, 67, 67, 67, 6~
```

```
## $ msbpr   <dbl> 135.0, 105.0, 91.0, 117.0, 102.0, 124.0, 120.0, 85.0, 112.0, ~
## $ mdbpr   <dbl> 80.0, 58.0, 60.0, 68.5, 78.0, 65.5, 77.0, 60.0, 74.0, 52.0, 1~
## $ hba1c   <dbl> 5.2, 5.3, 4.8, 4.8, 5.1, 5.1, 4.8, 4.9, 5.6, 4.2, 5.1, 5.3, 4~
## $ fbs     <dbl> 3.99, 4.26, 4.94, 4.60, 4.60, 4.42, 3.82, 4.40, 4.80, 3.68, 6~
## $ mogtt1h <dbl> 7.06, 8.63, 6.26, 4.31, 9.49, 6.29, NA, 6.43, 9.23, 6.70, 8.7~
## $ mogtt2h <dbl> 3.22, 6.49, 5.15, 3.85, 7.71, 5.65, 5.88, 4.89, 4.29, 2.59, 7~
## $ totchol <dbl> 5.43, 5.13, 5.55, 4.01, 5.21, 6.19, 4.33, 5.84, 6.14, 6.02, 6~
## $ ftrigliz <dbl> 1.06, 1.17, 0.72, 1.12, 0.78, 1.11, 0.73, 0.79, 1.63, 0.81, 1~
## $ hdl     <dbl> 1.65, 1.59, 2.24, 1.21, 1.43, 2.18, 0.98, 1.81, 1.63, 1.47, 1~
## $ ldl     <dbl> 2.69, 2.79, 2.55, 1.83, 2.40, 2.93, 1.82, 3.43, 3.71, 2.77, 3~
## $ gender  <chr> "female", "male", "female", "male", "female", "female", "fema~
## $ crural  <chr> "rural", "rural", "rural", "rural", "rural", "rural", "rural"~
```

9.6.4 Data wrangling

We will

- select only variable fbs, totchol, hpt and weight
- convert all character variables to factor variables
- then take a glance of the updated ms dataset again

```
ms <- ms %>%
  select(fbs, totchol, hpt , weight) %>%
  mutate(across(where(is.labelled), as_factor))
glimpse(ms)
```

```
## Rows: 4,340
## Columns: 4
## $ fbs     <dbl> 3.99, 4.26, 4.94, 4.60, 4.60, 4.42, 3.82, 4.40, 4.80, 3.68, 6.~
## $ totchol <dbl> 5.43, 5.13, 5.55, 4.01, 5.21, 6.19, 4.33, 5.84, 6.14, 6.02, 6.~
## $ hpt     <chr> "yes", "no", "no", "no", "no", "no", "no", "no", "no", "no", "~
## $ weight  <dbl> 40.0, 54.6, 37.0, 48.4, 44.5, 45.5, 48.0, 40.0, 48.4, 41.0, 52~
```

9.6.5 Create new categorical variable from fbs

Let us create a categorical (also known as a factor variable) based on this classification:

1. Normal if fbs is less than 6.1 mmol/L
2. Impaired Fasting Glucose (IFG) if fbs is between 6.1 mmol/L to 6.9 mmol/L
3. Diabetis Mellitus (DM) if fbs is 7.00 mmol/L or higher

```
ms <- ms %>%
  mutate(cat_fbs = cut(fbs,
                       breaks = c(2.50 , 6.10 , 6.90 , 28.01 ),
                       labels = c("Normal","IFG", "DM")))
ms %>%
  count(cat_fbs)
```

```
## # A tibble: 4 x 2
##   cat_fbs      n
##   <fct>    <int>
## 1 Normal    3130
## 2 IFG        364
## 3 DM         595
## 4 <NA>       251
```

We notice that there were 250 data has no values recorded as NA. Thus, we decide to remove observations when there are missing values for variable cat_fbs.

```
ms <- ms %>%
  filter(!is.na(cat_fbs))
ms %>%
  count(cat_fbs)
```

```
## # A tibble: 3 x 2
##   cat_fbs      n
##   <fct>    <int>
## 1 Normal    3130
## 2 IFG        364
## 3 DM         595
```

9.6.6 Exploratory data analysis

Next, is to return the table of summary statistics

```
ms %>%
  tbl_summary(by = cat_fbs,
              statistic = list(all_continuous() ~ "{mean} ({sd})",
                               all_categorical() ~ "{n} ({p}%)"),
              type = list(where(is.logical) ~ "categorical"),
              label = list(fbs ~ "Fasting Blood Sugar (mmol/L)",
                           totchol ~ "Total Cholesterol (mmol/L)",
↳ hpt~"Hypertension", weight ~ "Weight (kg)"),
```

```
            missing_text = "Missing") %>%
  modify_caption("**Table 1. Survey Participant Characteristic**")  %>%
  modify_header(label ~ "**Variable**") %>%
  modify_spanning_header(c("stat_1", "stat_2", "stat_3") ~ "**Glycemic Control
  ↪  Status**") %>%
  modify_footnote(all_stat_cols() ~ "Mean (SD) or Frequency (%)") %>%
  bold_labels() %>%
  as_gt()
```

	Glycemic Control Status		
Variable	**Normal**, N = 3,130[1]	**IFG**, N = 364[1]	**DM**, N = 595[1]
Fasting Blood Sugar (mmol/L)	4.76 (0.82)	6.44 (0.22)	10.41 (3.63)
Total Cholesterol (mmol/L)	5.69 (1.24)	6.08 (1.37)	6.16 (1.31)
Missing	4	0	1
Hypertension	281 (9.0%)	75 (21%)	126 (21%)
Weight (kg)	63 (14)	68 (14)	68 (15)
Missing	1	0	0

[1]Mean (SD) or Frequency (%)

9.6.7 Confirm the order of cat_fbs

```
levels(ms$cat_fbs)
```

```
## [1] "Normal" "IFG"    "DM"
```

However, we would like the DM as the smallest category. To do that we will use the
fct_relevel() function.

```
ms <- ms %>%
  mutate(cat_fbs = fct_relevel(cat_fbs,
                           c("DM", 'IFG', 'Normal')))
levels(ms$cat_fbs)
```

```
## [1] "DM"     "IFG"    "Normal"
```

9.7 Estimation

Our intention to investigate the relationship between totchol, hpt and weight with the outcome variables cat_fbs. Thus, we will perform multinomial logistic regression model to estimate the relation for 2 models:

- Model 1: DM vs Normal
- Model 2: IFG vs Normal

In both models, the reference group is Normal

9.7.1 Single independent variable

For independent variable totchol

```
log_chol <- vglm(cat_fbs ~ totchol,
                  multinomial, data = ms)
summary(log_chol)
```

```
##
## Call:
## vglm(formula = cat_fbs ~ totchol, family = multinomial, data = ms)
##
## Coefficients:
##                Estimate Std. Error z value Pr(>|z|)
## (Intercept):1  -3.33584    0.21306 -15.656  < 2e-16 ***
## (Intercept):2  -3.59935    0.25764 -13.970  < 2e-16 ***
## totchol:1       0.28357    0.03446   8.229  < 2e-16 ***
## totchol:2       0.24661    0.04176   5.905 3.53e-09 ***
## ---
## Signif. codes:  0 '***' 0.001 '**' 0.01 '*' 0.05 '.' 0.1 ' ' 1
##
## Names of linear predictors: log(mu[,1]/mu[,3]), log(mu[,2]/mu[,3])
##
## Residual deviance: 5634.468 on 8164 degrees of freedom
##
## Log-likelihood: -2817.234 on 8164 degrees of freedom
##
## Number of Fisher scoring iterations: 4
##
## Warning: Hauck-Donner effect detected in the following estimate(s):
## '(Intercept):2'
##
```

```
##
## Reference group is level  3  of the response
```

This is the model where hpt is the independent variable

```
log_hpt <- vglm(cat_fbs ~ hpt,
                multinomial, data = ms)
summary(log_hpt)
```

```
##
## Call:
## vglm(formula = cat_fbs ~ hpt, family = multinomial, data = ms)
##
## Coefficients:
##                 Estimate Std. Error z value Pr(>|z|)
## (Intercept):1 -1.80412    0.04983 -36.205  < 2e-16 ***
## (Intercept):2 -2.28830    0.06173 -37.067  < 2e-16 ***
## hptyes:1       1.00205    0.11823   8.475  < 2e-16 ***
## hptyes:2       0.96743    0.14389   6.724 1.77e-11 ***
## ---
## Signif. codes:  0 '***' 0.001 '**' 0.01 '*' 0.05 '.' 0.1 ' ' 1
##
## Names of linear predictors: log(mu[,1]/mu[,3]), log(mu[,2]/mu[,3])
##
## Residual deviance: 5637.16 on 8174 degrees of freedom
##
## Log-likelihood: -2818.58 on 8174 degrees of freedom
##
## Number of Fisher scoring iterations: 4
##
## No Hauck-Donner effect found in any of the estimates
##
##
## Reference group is level  3  of the response
```

And lastly, the independent variable is weight

```
log_wt <- vglm(cat_fbs ~ weight,
               multinomial, data = ms)
summary(log_wt)
```

```
##
## Call:
## vglm(formula = cat_fbs ~ weight, family = multinomial, data = ms)
##
```

```
## Coefficients:
##                 Estimate Std. Error z value Pr(>|z|)
## (Intercept):1 -3.214303    0.204303 -15.733  < 2e-16 ***
## (Intercept):2 -3.672632    0.249121 -14.742  < 2e-16 ***
## weight:1       0.023860    0.002988   7.984 1.42e-15 ***
## weight:2       0.023372    0.003627   6.444 1.16e-10 ***
## ---
## Signif. codes:  0 '***' 0.001 '**' 0.01 '*' 0.05 '.' 0.1 ' ' 1
##
## Names of linear predictors: log(mu[,1]/mu[,3]), log(mu[,2]/mu[,3])
##
## Residual deviance: 5638.998 on 8172 degrees of freedom
##
## Log-likelihood: -2819.499 on 8172 degrees of freedom
##
## Number of Fisher scoring iterations: 4
##
## Warning: Hauck-Donner effect detected in the following estimate(s):
## '(Intercept):2'
##
##
## Reference group is level  3  of the response
```

9.7.2   Multiple independent variables

We feel that totchol, hpt and weight are all important independent variables. Hence, we want to fit a model with the three independent variables as the covariates.

```
mlog <- vglm(cat_fbs ~ totchol + hpt + weight,
             multinomial, data = ms)
summary(mlog)
```

```
##
## Call:
## vglm(formula = cat_fbs ~ totchol + hpt + weight, family = multinomial,
##     data = ms)
##
## Coefficients:
##                 Estimate Std. Error z value Pr(>|z|)
## (Intercept):1 -4.907874    0.303768 -16.157  < 2e-16 ***
## (Intercept):2 -5.112990    0.366325 -13.958  < 2e-16 ***
## totchol:1      0.277217    0.035055   7.908 2.62e-15 ***
## totchol:2      0.239413    0.042391   5.648 1.63e-08 ***
## hptyes:1       0.899987    0.120451   7.472 7.91e-14 ***
```

```
## hptyes:2        0.867136   0.145569   5.957 2.57e-09 ***
## weight:1        0.022678   0.003074   7.378 1.61e-13 ***
## weight:2        0.021994   0.003710   5.928 3.07e-09 ***
## ---
## Signif. codes:  0 '***' 0.001 '**' 0.01 '*' 0.05 '.' 0.1 ' ' 1
##
## Names of linear predictors: log(mu[,1]/mu[,3]), log(mu[,2]/mu[,3])
##
## Residual deviance: 5476.397 on 8158 degrees of freedom
##
## Log-likelihood: -2738.199 on 8158 degrees of freedom
##
## Number of Fisher scoring iterations: 5
##
## Warning: Hauck-Donner effect detected in the following estimate(s):
## '(Intercept):1', '(Intercept):2'
##
##
## Reference group is level  3  of the response
```

9.7.3   Model with interaction term between independent variables

Then, we hypothesize that there could be a significant interaction between totchol and weight. And to test the hypothesis, we extend the multivariable logistic regression model by adding an interaction term. This interaction term is a product between variable weight and totchol.

```
mlogi <- vglm(cat_fbs ~ totchol + hpt + weight + totchol*weight,
              multinomial, data = ms)
summary(mlogi)


##
## Call:
## vglm(formula = cat_fbs ~ totchol + hpt + weight + totchol * weight,
##      family = multinomial, data = ms)
##
## Coefficients:
##                  Estimate Std. Error z value Pr(>|z|)
## (Intercept):1  -5.1253325  0.9671480  -5.299 1.16e-07 ***
## (Intercept):2  -7.0506874  1.1195704  -6.298 3.02e-10 ***
## totchol:1       0.3155740  0.1605324   1.966  0.04932 *
## totchol:2       0.5747241  0.1878902   3.059  0.00222 **
## hptyes:1        0.8984459  0.1204877   7.457 8.87e-14 ***
## hptyes:2        0.8643701  0.1455478   5.939 2.87e-09 ***
```

```
## weight:1            0.0260899  0.0142834   1.827  0.06776 .
## weight:2            0.0514503  0.0165054   3.117  0.00183 **
## totchol:weight:1 -0.0006015  0.0023804  -0.253  0.80052
## totchol:weight:2 -0.0051091  0.0028023  -1.823  0.06828 .
## ---
## Signif. codes:  0 '***' 0.001 '**' 0.01 '*' 0.05 '.' 0.1 ' ' 1
##
## Names of linear predictors: log(mu[,1]/mu[,3]), log(mu[,2]/mu[,3])
##
## Residual deviance: 5473.004 on 8156 degrees of freedom
##
## Log-likelihood: -2736.502 on 8156 degrees of freedom
##
## Number of Fisher scoring iterations: 5
##
## Warning: Hauck-Donner effect detected in the following estimate(s):
## '(Intercept):1', '(Intercept):2'
##
##
## Reference group is level  3  of the response
```

The interaction term in our model showed p-values above 0.05 (p-values of 0.80 and 0.07, respectively). As the p-value is bigger than the level of significance at 5% and the value of regression parameters for the interaction terms are likely not clinically meaningful, we have decided not to use the model with an interaction term.

9.8   Inferences

For the inference, we will

- calculate the 95% CI (interval estimates)
- calculate the p-values (hypothesis testing)

There is no facility inside the broom::tidy() function to generate confidence intervals for object with class vglm. Because of that we will use the coef(), confint() and cind(0 functions to produce a rather nice table of inferences.

We are going to follow these steps:

- set the number of digits equal to 2 to limit the decimal numbers
- return the regression coefficents for all $\hat{\beta}$ as an object named b_fitmlog2
- return the confidence intervals for all $\hat{\beta}$ as an object named ci_fitmlog2
- combine the $\hat{\beta}$ and the corresponding 95% CIs

TABLE 9.1

Log odds from multinomial logistic regression

	log odds	Lower CI	Upper CI
(Intercept):1	−4.91	−5.50	−4.31
(Intercept):2	−5.11	−5.83	−4.40
totchol:1	0.28	0.21	0.35
totchol:2	0.24	0.16	0.32
hptyes:1	0.90	0.66	1.14
hptyes:2	0.87	0.58	1.15
weight:1	0.02	0.02	0.03
weight:2	0.02	0.01	0.03

TABLE 9.2

Log odds and RRR from multinomial logistic regression

	b	lower b	upper b	RRR	lower RRR	upper RRR
(Intercept):1	−4.91	−5.50	−4.31	0.01	0.00	0.01
(Intercept):2	−5.11	−5.83	−4.40	0.01	0.00	0.01
totchol:1	0.28	0.21	0.35	1.32	1.23	1.41
totchol:2	0.24	0.16	0.32	1.27	1.17	1.38
hptyes:1	0.90	0.66	1.14	2.46	1.94	3.11
hptyes:2	0.87	0.58	1.15	2.38	1.79	3.17
weight:1	0.02	0.02	0.03	1.02	1.02	1.03
weight:2	0.02	0.01	0.03	1.02	1.01	1.03

```
b_mlog <- coef(mlog)
ci_mlog <- confint(mlog)
b_ci_mlog <- data.frame(b_mlog,ci_mlog) %>%
  rename("log odds" = b_mlog, "Lower CI" = X2.5.., "Upper CI" = X97.5..)
b_ci_mlog %>%
  kbl(digits = 2, booktabs = T, caption = "Log odds from multinomial logistic
  ↳ regression") %>%
  kable_styling(position = "center")
```

Afterwards, we will *exponentiate* the coefficients to obtain the **relative-risk ratio**. We then combine the results to the previous table. Finally, we will name the columns of the object `tab_fitmlog2`.

```
rrr_mlog <- exp(b_ci_mlog)
tab_mlog <- cbind(b_ci_mlog, rrr_mlog)
colnames(tab_mlog) <- c('b', 'lower b', 'upper b',
                        'RRR', 'lower RRR', 'upper RRR')
tab_mlog %>%
  kbl(digits = 2, booktabs = T, caption = "Log odds and RRR from multinomial
  ↪ logistic regression") %>%
  kable_styling(position = "center")
```

9.9   Interpretation

The result from our multivariable logistic regression models can be interpreted as below:

- Every increment 1 mmol/L of totchol (Total cholesterol) when controlling for hypertension status and weight; a) the odds of being in DM group (in comparison to Normal) change by 0.277 (Adjusted RRR = 1.32, 95% CI : 1.232, 1.413, p-value <0.001) and b) the odds of being in IFG group (in comparison to being in Normal) change by 0.239 (Adjusted RRR = 1.27, 95% CI : 1.169,1.381, p-value <0.001).
- Every increment 1 kg of weight when controlling for hypertension status and total cholesterol; a) the odds of being in DM group (in comparison to being in Normal) increase by 0.023 (Adjusted RRR = 1.02, 95% CI : 1.017,1.029, p-value <0.001), and b) the odds of being in IFG group (in comparison being in Normal) increase by 0.022 (Adjusted RRR = 1.02, 95% CI : 1.015,1.030, p-value <0.001).
- In the population with hypertension (as compared with participant without hypertension) when controlling for weight and total cholesterol; a) their odds of being in DM group (in comparison to being in Normal) change by 0.900 (Adjusted RRR = 2.5, 95% CI : 1.942, 3.114, p-value <0.001). When repeated research on this population, the odds ranging between reduced the odds by 0.481 to 0.677, and b) and their odds of being in IFG group (in comparison to being Normal) change by 0.867 (Adjusted RRR = 2.38, 95% CI : 1.789, 3.166, p-value <0.001).

9.10   Prediction

We can calculate the predicted probability of each category of outcome by using the `predict()` function. Below are the result for the top 10 observations.

```
predict.vgam(mlog, type = 'response') %>%
  head(10)
```

```
##             DM        IFG    Normal
## 1   0.15254733 0.09528434 0.7521683
## 2   0.09000250 0.05817369 0.8518238
## 3   0.07042058 0.04534241 0.8842370
## 4   0.06047226 0.04095046 0.8985773
## 5   0.07525337 0.04882982 0.8759168
## 6   0.09712040 0.06068516 0.8421944
## 7   0.06497274 0.04348092 0.8915463
## 8   0.08025639 0.05100727 0.8687363
## 9   0.10144228 0.06337974 0.8351780
## 10  0.08548801 0.05392687 0.8605851
```

9.11 Presentation of Multinomial Regression Model

We can make a *better* table using **knitr** and **kableExtra** packages. Or we can save the results as a .csv file so we can edit it using spreadsheets.

```
tab_mlog %>%
  write_csv("results_multinomial.csv")
```

9.12 Summary

In this chapter, we extend binary logistic regression analysis to data with a categorical outcome variable that has three or more levels. We describe the multinomial logistic regression model, the log odds and also the conditional probabilities. When then show estimation for the single and multiple multinomial logistic regression including models with an interaction. Following that, we describe how to make inferences and perform predictions. Lastly, we make use of **kableExtra** package to produce a nice table for our model. We are big fans of two excellent books on logistic regression. The first one is Applied Logistic Regression (Hosmer et al., 2013) and the second one is Logistic Regression: Self Learning Text (Kleinbaum, 2010). You will acquire strong understanding of the concepts and model-building process from the two books. To see what packages and functions relevant to logistic regression, you can refer to A Handbook of Statistical Analyses Using R (Everitt and Hothorn, 2017).

10

Poisson Regression

10.1 Objectives

After completing this chapter, the readers are expected to

- understand the basic concepts behind Poisson regression for count and rate data
- perform Poisson regression for count and rate
- perform model fit assessment
- present and interpret the results of Poisson regression analyses

10.2 Introduction

Poisson regression is a regression analysis for count and rate data. As mentioned before in Chapter 7, it is a type of generalized linear models (GLMs) whenever the outcome is count. It also accommodates rate data, as we will see shortly. Although count and rate data are very common in medical and health sciences, in our experience, Poisson regression is underutilized in medical research. Most often, researchers end up using linear regression because they are more familiar with it and lack of exposure to the advantage of using Poisson regression to handle count and rate data.

Count is discrete numerical data. Although it is convenient to use linear regression to handle the count outcome by assuming the count or *discrete* numerical data (e.g. the number of hospital admissions) as *continuous* numerical data (e.g. systolic blood pressure in mmHg), it may result in illogical predicted values. For example, by using linear regression to predict the number of asthmatic attacks in the past one year, we may end up with a negative number of attacks, which does not make any clinical sense! So, it is recommended that medical researchers get familiar with Poisson regression and make use of it whenever the outcome variable is a count variable.

Another reason for using Poisson regression is whenever the number of cases (e.g. deaths and accidents) is small relative to the number of no events (e.g. alive and no accident), then it makes more sense to just get the information from the cases in a population of interest, instead of also getting the information from the non-cases as in typical cohort and case-control studies. For example, in the publicly available COVID-19 data, only the number of deaths were reported along with some basic sociodemographic and clinical information for the cases. Whenever the information for the non-cases are available, it is quite easy to instead use logistic regression for the analysis.

Basically, Poisson regression models the linear relationship between:

- **outcome**: count variable (e.g. the number of hospital admissions, parity, cancerous lesions and asthmatic attacks). This is transformed into the natural log scale.
- **predictors/independent variables**: numerical variables (e.g. age, blood pressure and income) and categorical variables (e.g. gender, race and education level).

We might be interested in knowing the relationship between the number of asthmatic attacks in the past one year with sociodemographic factors. This relationship can be explored by a Poisson regression analysis.

Basically, for Poisson regression, the relationship between the outcome and predictors is as follows,

$$natural\ log\ of\ count\ outcome = numerical\ predictors \\ + categorical\ predictors$$

At times, the count is proportional to a denominator. For example, given the same number of deaths, the death rate in a small population will be higher than the rate in a large population. If we were to compare the number of deaths between the populations, it would not make a fair comparison. Thus, we may consider adding denominators in the Poisson regression modeling in the form of offsets. This denominator could also be the unit time of exposure, for example person-years of cigarette smoking. This will be explained later under Poisson regression for rate section.

In the previous chapter, we learned that logistic regression allows us to obtain the odds ratio, which is approximately the relative risk given a predictor. For Poisson regression, by taking the exponent of the coefficient, we obtain the *rate ratio* RR (also known as *incidence rate ratio* IRR),

$$RR = exp(b_p)$$

for the coefficient b_p of the p's predictor. This is interpreted in similar way to the odds ratio for logistic regression, which is approximately the relative risk given a predictor.

10.3   Prepare R Environment for Analysis

10.3.1   Libraries

For this chapter, we will be using the following packages:

- **tidyverse**: a general and powerful package for data transformation
- **psych**: for descriptive statistics
- **gtsummary**: for coming up with nice tables for results
- **broom**: for tidying up the results
- **epiDisplay**: an epidemiological data display package

These are loaded as follows using the function `library()`,

```
library(tidyverse)
library(psych)
library(gtsummary)
library(broom)
```

For `epiDisplay`, we will use the package directly using `epiDisplay::function_name()` instead. We did not load the package as we usually do with `library(epiDisplay)` because it has some conflicts with the packages we loaded above.

10.4   Poisson Regression for Count

10.4.1   About Poisson regression for count

Poisson regression models the linear relationship between:

- **outcome**: count variable (e.g. the number of hospital admissions, parity, cancerous lesions and asthmatic attacks). This is transformed into the natural log scale.
- **predictor(s)**: numerical variables (e.g. age, blood pressure and income) and categorical variables (e.g. gender, race and education level).

We might be interested in knowing the relationship between the number of asthmatic attacks in the past one year with sociodemographic factors. This relationship can be explored by a Poisson regression analysis.

Multiple Poisson regression for count is given as,

$$ln(count\ outcome) = intercept$$
$$+ coefficients \times numerical\ predictors$$
$$+ coefficients \times categorical\ predictors$$

or in a shorter form,

$$ln(\hat{y}) = b_0 + b_1 x_1 + b_2 x_2 + ... + b_p x_p$$

where we have p predictors.

10.4.2   Dataset

The data on the number of asthmatic attacks per year among a sample of 120 patients and the associated factors are given in `asthma.csv`.

The dataset contains four variables:

1. *gender*: Gender of the subjects (categorical) {male, female}.
2. *res_inf*: Recurrent respiratory infection (categorical) {no, yes}.
3. *ghq12*: General Health Questionnare 12 (GHQ-12) score of psychological well being (numerical) {0 to 36}.
4. *attack*: Number of athmatic attack per year (count).

The dataset is loaded as follows,

```
asthma = read.csv("data/asthma.csv")
```

We then look at the basic structure of the dataset,

```
str(asthma)
```

```
## 'data.frame':    120 obs. of  4 variables:
## $ gender : chr  "female" "male" "male" "female" ...
## $ res_inf: chr  "yes" "no" "yes" "yes" ...
## $ ghq12  : int  21 17 30 22 27 33 24 23 25 28 ...
## $ attack : int  6 4 8 5 2 3 2 1 2 2 ...
```

10.4.3   Data exploration

For descriptive statistics, we introduce the `epidisplay` package. It is a nice package that allows us to easily obtain statistics for both numerical and categorical variables at the same time. We use `codebook()` function from the package.

```
epiDisplay::codebook(asthma)
```

```
##
##
```

```
##
## gender    :
## A character vector
##
##   ==================
## res_inf   :
## A character vector
##
##   ==================
## ghq12     :
##  obs. mean   median  s.d.   min.   max.
##  120  16.342 19       9.81   0      33
##
##   ==================
## attack    :
##  obs. mean   median  s.d.   min.   max.
##  120  2.458  2        2.012  0      9
##
##   ==================
```

10.4.4 Univariable analysis

For the univariable analysis, we fit univariable Poisson regression models for gender (gender), recurrent respiratory infection (res_inf) and GHQ12 (ghq12) variables.

```
# gender
pois_attack1 = glm(attack ~ gender, data = asthma, family = "poisson")
summary(pois_attack1)
```

```
##
## Call:
## glm(formula = attack ~ gender, family = "poisson", data = asthma)
##
## Deviance Residuals:
##      Min        1Q    Median        3Q       Max
## -2.35632  -1.22887  -0.03965   0.68859   3.13805
##
## Coefficients:
##              Estimate Std. Error z value Pr(>|z|)
## (Intercept)   1.02105    0.07332  13.925   <2e-16 ***
## gendermale   -0.30000    0.12063  -2.487   0.0129 *
## ---
## Signif. codes:  0 '***' 0.001 '**' 0.01 '*' 0.05 '.' 0.1 ' ' 1
##
```

```
## (Dispersion parameter for poisson family taken to be 1)
##
##      Null deviance: 229.56  on 119   degrees of freedom
## Residual deviance: 223.23  on 118   degrees of freedom
## AIC: 500.3
##
## Number of Fisher Scoring iterations: 5
```

```
# rec_res_inf
pois_attack2 = glm(attack ~ res_inf, data = asthma, family = "poisson")
summary(pois_attack2)
```

```
##
## Call:
## glm(formula = attack ~ res_inf, family = "poisson", data = asthma)
##
## Deviance Residuals:
##      Min       1Q    Median       3Q       Max
## -2.5651  -1.4826   -0.1622    0.6216    2.9522
##
## Coefficients:
##              Estimate Std. Error z value Pr(>|z|)
## (Intercept)    0.2877     0.1213   2.372   0.0177 *
## res_infyes     0.9032     0.1382   6.533 6.44e-11 ***
## ---
## Signif. codes:  0 '***' 0.001 '**' 0.01 '*' 0.05 '.' 0.1 ' ' 1
##
## (Dispersion parameter for poisson family taken to be 1)
##
##      Null deviance: 229.56  on 119   degrees of freedom
## Residual deviance: 180.49  on 118   degrees of freedom
## AIC: 457.56
##
## Number of Fisher Scoring iterations: 5
```

```
# ghq12
pois_attack3 = glm(attack ~ ghq12, data = asthma, family = "poisson")
summary(pois_attack3)
```

```
##
## Call:
## glm(formula = attack ~ ghq12, family = "poisson", data = asthma)
##
## Deviance Residuals:
```

```
##      Min       1Q   Median       3Q      Max
## -2.0281  -1.2600  -0.1511   0.7060   2.3061
##
## Coefficients:
##               Estimate Std. Error z value Pr(>|z|)
## (Intercept) -0.230923   0.159128  -1.451    0.147
## ghq12        0.059500   0.006919   8.599   <2e-16 ***
## ---
## Signif. codes:  0 '***' 0.001 '**' 0.01 '*' 0.05 '.' 0.1 ' ' 1
##
## (Dispersion parameter for poisson family taken to be 1)
##
##     Null deviance: 229.56  on 119  degrees of freedom
## Residual deviance: 145.13  on 118  degrees of freedom
## AIC: 422.2
##
## Number of Fisher Scoring iterations: 5
```

From the outputs, all variables are important with $p < .25$. These variables are the candidates for inclusion in the multivariable analysis. However, as a reminder, in the context of **confirmatory research**, the variables that we want to include must consider expert judgment.

10.4.5 Multivariable analysis

For the multivariable analysis, we included all variables as predictors of `attack`. Here we use dot . as a shortcut for all variables when specifying the right-hand side of the formula of the `glm`.

```
pois_attack_all = glm(attack ~ ., data = asthma, family = "poisson")
summary(pois_attack_all)
```

```
##
## Call:
## glm(formula = attack ~ ., family = "poisson", data = asthma)
##
## Deviance Residuals:
##      Min       1Q   Median       3Q      Max
## -2.0734  -1.2125  -0.2297   0.7274   2.3949
##
## Coefficients:
##               Estimate Std. Error z value Pr(>|z|)
## (Intercept) -0.315387   0.183500  -1.719  0.08566 .
## gendermale  -0.041905   0.122469  -0.342  0.73222
## res_infyes   0.426431   0.152859   2.790  0.00528 **
```

```
## ghq12         0.049508    0.007878    6.285 3.29e-10 ***
## ---
## Signif. codes:  0 '***' 0.001 '**' 0.01 '*' 0.05 '.' 0.1 ' ' 1
##
## (Dispersion parameter for poisson family taken to be 1)
##
##      Null deviance: 229.56  on 119   degrees of freedom
## Residual deviance: 136.68  on 116   degrees of freedom
## AIC: 417.75
##
## Number of Fisher Scoring iterations: 5
```

From the output, we noted that gender is not significant with $p > 0.05$, although it was significant at the univariable analysis. Now, we fit a model excluding gender,

```
# minus gender
pois_attack_all1 = glm(attack ~ res_inf + ghq12, data = asthma,
                        family = "poisson")
summary(pois_attack_all1)
```

```
##
## Call:
## glm(formula = attack ~ res_inf + ghq12, family = "poisson", data = asthma)
##
## Deviance Residuals:
##     Min      1Q   Median      3Q      Max
## -2.0514  -1.2229  -0.2033   0.7041   2.4257
##
## Coefficients:
##              Estimate Std. Error z value Pr(>|z|)
## (Intercept) -0.34051    0.16823   -2.024  0.04296 *
## res_infyes   0.42816    0.15282    2.802  0.00508 **
## ghq12        0.04989    0.00779    6.404 1.51e-10 ***
## ---
## Signif. codes:  0 '***' 0.001 '**' 0.01 '*' 0.05 '.' 0.1 ' ' 1
##
## (Dispersion parameter for poisson family taken to be 1)
##
##      Null deviance: 229.56  on 119   degrees of freedom
## Residual deviance: 136.80  on 117   degrees of freedom
## AIC: 415.86
##
## Number of Fisher Scoring iterations: 5
```

From the output, both variables are significant predictors of asthmatic attack (or more accurately the natural log of the count of asthmatic attack). This serves as our **preliminary model**.

10.4.6 Interaction

Now, we include a two-way interaction term between `res_inf` and `ghq12`.

```
pois_attack_allx = glm(attack ~ res_inf * ghq12, data = asthma,
                       family = "poisson")
summary(pois_attack_allx)
```

```
##
## Call:
## glm(formula = attack ~ res_inf * ghq12, family = "poisson", data = asthma)
##
## Deviance Residuals:
##     Min      1Q   Median      3Q      Max
## -2.0626  -1.0656  -0.2430   0.6169   2.3274
##
## Coefficients:
##                    Estimate Std. Error z value Pr(>|z|)
## (Intercept)        -0.63436    0.23408  -2.710  0.00673 **
## res_infyes          1.01927    0.32822   3.105  0.00190 **
## ghq12               0.06834    0.01186   5.763 8.29e-09 ***
## res_infyes:ghq12   -0.03135    0.01531  -2.048  0.04056 *
## ---
## Signif. codes:  0 '***' 0.001 '**' 0.01 '*' 0.05 '.' 0.1 ' ' 1
##
## (Dispersion parameter for poisson family taken to be 1)
##
##     Null deviance: 229.56  on 119  degrees of freedom
## Residual deviance: 132.67  on 116  degrees of freedom
## AIC: 413.74
##
## Number of Fisher Scoring iterations: 5
```

It turns out that the interaction term `res_inf * ghq12` is significant. We may include this interaction term in the final model. However, this might complicate our interpretation of the result as we can no longer interpret individual coefficients. Given that the *p*-value of the interaction term is close to the commonly used significance level of 0.05, we may choose to ignore this interaction. But keep in mind that the decision is yours, the analyst. Having said that, if the purpose of modeling is mainly for prediction, the issue is less severe because we are more concerned with the predicted values than with the clinical interpretation of the result. However, if you insist on including the interaction, it can be done by writing down the equation for the model, substitute the value of `res_inf` with yes = 1 or no = 0, and obtain the coefficient for `ghq12`. We will see how to do this under **Presentation and interpretation** below.

10.4.7 Model fit assessment

For Poisson regression, we assess the model fit by chi-square goodness-of-fit test, model-to-model AIC comparison and scaled Pearson chi-square statistic. We also assess the regression diagnostics using standardized residuals.

Chi-square goodness-of-fit

Chi-square goodness-of-fit test can be performed using `poisgof()` function in `epiDisplay` package. Note that, instead of using Pearson chi-square statistic, it utilizes residual deviance with its respective degrees of freedom (df) (e.g. from the output of `summary(pois_attack_all1)` above). A p-value > 0.05 indicates good model fit.

```
epiDisplay::poisgof(pois_attack_all1)
```

```
## $results
## [1] "Goodness-of-fit test for Poisson assumption"
##
## $chisq
## [1] 136.7964
##
## $df
## [1] 117
##
## $p.value
## [1] 0.101934
```

Model-to-model AIC comparison

We may also compare the models that we fit so far by Akaike information criterion (AIC). Recall that R uses AIC for stepwise automatic variable selection, which was explained in Linear Regression chapter.

```
AIC(pois_attack1, pois_attack2, pois_attack3,
    pois_attack_all1, pois_attack_allx)
```

```
##                   df      AIC
## pois_attack1       2 500.3009
## pois_attack2       2 457.5555
## pois_attack3       2 422.1997
## pois_attack_all1   3 415.8649
## pois_attack_allx   4 413.7424
```

The best model is the one with the lowest AIC, which is the model model with the interaction term. However, since the model with the interaction term differ slightly from the model without interaction, we may instead choose the simpler model without the interaction term.

Scaled Pearson chi-square statistic

Pearson chi-square statistic divided by its *df* gives rise to scaled Pearson chi-square statistic (Fleiss et al., 2003). The closer the value of this statistic to 1, the better is the model fit. First, Pearson chi-square statistic is calculated as,

$$\chi_P^2 = \sum_{i=1}^{n} \frac{(y_i - \hat{y}_i)^2}{\hat{y}_i}$$

easily obtained in R as below.

```
x2 = sum((asthma$attack - pois_attack_all1$fitted)^2 /
         pois_attack_all1$fitted)
```

Then we obtain scaled Pearson chi-square statistic χ_P^2/df, where $df = n - p$. n is the number of observations nrow(asthma) and p is the number of coefficients/parameters we estimated for the model length(pois_attack_all1$coefficients).

```
df = nrow(asthma) - length(pois_attack_all1$coefficients)
sx2 = x2 / df; sx2
```

```
## [1] 1.052376
```

The value of sx2 is 1.052, which is close to 1. This indicates good model fit.

It is actually easier to obtain scaled Pearson chi-square by changing the family = "poisson" to family = "quasipoisson" in the glm specification, then viewing the dispersion value from the summary of the model. It works because scaled Pearson chi-square is an estimator of the overdispersion parameter in a quasi-Poisson regression model (Fleiss et al., 2003). We will discuss about quasi-Poisson regression later towards the end of this chapter.

```
qpois_attack_all1_summ = summary(glm(attack ~ res_inf + ghq12,
                          data = asthma, family = "quasipoisson"))
qpois_attack_all1_summ$dispersion
```

```
## [1] 1.052383
```

Regression diagnostics

Here, we use standardized residuals using `rstandard()` function. Because it is in form of standardized z score, we may use specific cutoffs to find the outliers, for example 1.96 (for $\alpha = 0.05$) or 3.89 (for $\alpha = 0.0001$).

```
std_res = rstandard(pois_attack_all1)
std_res[abs(std_res) > 1.96]
```

```
##         28         38         95        103
## -2.082287   2.168737   1.977013   2.461419
```

We now locate where the discrepancies are,

```
index = names(std_res[abs(std_res) > 1.96])
cbind(asthma[index,], attack_pred = pois_attack_all1$fitted[index])
```

```
##        gender res_inf ghq12 attack attack_pred
## 28     female     yes    29      1   4.6384274
## 38     female     yes    26      9   3.9936854
## 95       male      no     1      3   0.7477996
## 103    female      no    19      6   1.8355524
```

10.4.8   Presentation and interpretation

Model without interaction

After all these assumption check points, we decide on the final model and rename the model for easier reference.

```
pois_attack_final = pois_attack_all1
```

We use `tbl_regression()` to come up with a table for the results. Here, for interpretation, we exponentiate the coefficients to obtain the incidence rate ratio, *IRR*.

```
tbl_regression(pois_attack_final, exponentiate = TRUE)
```

Characteristic	IRR[1]	95% CI[1]	p-value
res_inf			
no	—	—	
yes	1.53	1.14, 2.08	0.005
ghq12	1.05	1.04, 1.07	< 0.001

[1]IRR = Incidence Rate Ratio, CI = Confidence Interval

Based on this table, we may interpret the results as follows:

- Those with recurrent respiratory infection are at higher risk of having an asthmatic attack with an IRR of 1.53 (95% CI: 1.14, 2.08), while controlling for the effect of GHQ-12 score.
- An increase in GHQ-12 score by one mark increases the risk of having an asthmatic attack by 1.05 (95% CI: 1.04, 1.07), while controlling for the effect of recurrent respiratory infection.

We can also view and save the output in a format suitable for exporting to the spreadsheet format for later use. We use `tidy()` function for the job,

```
tib_pois_attack = tidy(pois_attack_final, exponentiate = TRUE,
                  conf.int = TRUE)
tib_pois_attack
```

```
## # A tibble: 3 x 7
##   term         estimate std.error statistic  p.value conf.low conf.high
##   <chr>           <dbl>     <dbl>     <dbl>    <dbl>    <dbl>     <dbl>
## 1 (Intercept)     0.711    0.168     -2.02  4.30e- 2    0.505     0.978
## 2 res_infyes      1.53     0.153      2.80  5.08e- 3    1.14      2.08
## 3 ghq12           1.05     0.00779    6.40  1.51e-10    1.04      1.07
```

and export it to a `.csv` file,

```
write.csv(tib_pois_attack, "tib_pois_attack.csv")
```

Then, we display the coefficients (i.e. without the exponent) and transfer the values into an equation,

```
round(summary(pois_attack_final)$coefficients, 2)
```

```
##              Estimate Std. Error z value Pr(>|z|)
## (Intercept)     -0.34       0.17   -2.02     0.04
## res_infyes       0.43       0.15    2.80     0.01
```

```
## ghq12          0.05        0.01     6.40        0.00
```

$$ln(attack) = -0.34 + 0.43 \times res\_inf + 0.05 \times ghq12$$

From the table and equation above, the effect of an increase in GHQ-12 score is by one mark might not be clinically of interest. Let say, as a clinician we want to know the effect of an increase in GHQ-12 score by six marks instead, which is 1/6 of the maximum score of 36. From the coefficient for GHQ-12 of 0.05, the risk is calculated as

$$IRR_{GHQ12\,by\,6} = exp(0.05 \times 6) = 1.35$$

Or we may fit the model again with some adjustment to the data and glm specification. First, we divide ghq12 values by 6 and save the values into a new variable ghq12_by6, followed by fitting the model again using the edited data set and new variable,

```
# Divide ghq12 by 6
asthma_new = asthma %>% mutate(ghq12_by6 = ghq12 / 6)
# Fit the model
pois_attack_final_by6 = glm(attack ~ res_inf + ghq12_by6,
                            data = asthma_new, family = "poisson")
```

Now we view the results for the re-fitted model,

```
# coeffients
tidy(pois_attack_final_by6, conf.int = TRUE)
```

```
## # A tibble: 3 x 7
##    term          estimate std.error statistic  p.value conf.low conf.high
##    <chr>            <dbl>    <dbl>     <dbl>    <dbl>    <dbl>    <dbl>
## 1 (Intercept)     -0.341    0.168    -2.02 4.30e- 2   -0.682   -0.0222
## 2 res_infyes       0.428    0.153     2.80 5.08e- 3    0.135    0.734
## 3 ghq12_by6        0.299    0.0467    6.40 1.51e-10    0.209    0.392
```

```
# IRRs
tidy(pois_attack_final_by6, exponentiate = TRUE, conf.int = TRUE)
```

```
## # A tibble: 3 x 7
##    term          estimate std.error statistic  p.value conf.low conf.high
##    <chr>            <dbl>    <dbl>     <dbl>    <dbl>    <dbl>    <dbl>
## 1 (Intercept)      0.711    0.168    -2.02 4.30e- 2    0.505    0.978
## 2 res_infyes       1.53     0.153     2.80 5.08e- 3    1.14     2.08
## 3 ghq12_by6        1.35     0.0467    6.40 1.51e-10    1.23     1.48
```

As compared to the first method that requires multiplying the coefficient manually, the second method is preferable in R as we also get the 95% CI for ghq12_by6.

Model with interaction

Now we will go through the interpretation of the model with interaction. We display the coefficients for the model with interaction (pois_attack_allx) and enter the values into an equation,

```
round(summary(pois_attack_allx)$coefficients, 2)
```

```
##                     Estimate Std. Error z value Pr(>|z|)
## (Intercept)           -0.63       0.23   -2.71     0.01
## res_infyes             1.02       0.33    3.11     0.00
## ghq12                  0.07       0.01    5.76     0.00
## res_infyes:ghq12      -0.03       0.02   -2.05     0.04
```

$$ln(attack) = -0.34 + 0.43 \times res\_inf + 0.05 \times ghq12$$
$$- 0.03 \times res\_inf \times ghq12$$

As we need to interpret the coefficient for ghq12 by the status of res_inf, we write an equation for each res_inf status. When res_inf = 1 (yes),

$$ln(attack) = -0.63 + 1.02 \times res\_inf + 0.07 \times ghq12$$
$$- 0.03 \times res\_inf \times ghq12$$
$$= -0.63 + 1.02 \times 1 + 0.07 \times ghq12 - 0.03 \times 1 \times ghq12$$
$$= 0.39 + 0.04 \times ghq12$$

and when res_inf = 0 (no),

$$ln(attack) = -0.63 + 1.02 \times res\_inf + 0.07 \times ghq12$$
$$- 0.03 \times res\_inf \times ghq12$$
$$= -0.63 + 1.02 \times 0 + 0.07 \times ghq12 - 0.03 \times 0 \times ghq12$$
$$= -0.63 + 0.07 \times ghq12$$

Now, based on the equations, we may interpret the results as follows:

- For those with recurrent respiratory infection, an increase in GHQ-12 score by one mark increases the risk of having an asthmatic attack by 1.04 (IRR = exp[0.04]).
- For those without recurrent respiratory infection, an increase in GHQ-12 score by one mark increases the risk of having an asthmatic attack by 1.07 (IRR = exp[0.07]).

Based on these IRRs, the effect of an increase of GHQ-12 score is slightly higher for those without recurrent respiratory infection. However, in comparison to the IRR for an increase in GHQ-12 score by one mark in the model without interaction, with

IRR = exp(0.05) = 1.05. So there are minimal differences in the IRR values for GHQ-12 between the models, thus in this case the simpler Poisson regression model without interaction is preferable. But now, you get the idea as to how to interpret the model with an interaction term.

10.4.9 Prediction

We can use the final model above for prediction. Relevant to our data set, we may want to know the expected number of asthmatic attacks per year for a patient with recurrent respiratory infection and GHQ-12 score of 8,

```
pred = predict(pois_attack_final, list(res_inf = "yes", ghq12 = 8),
               type = "response")
round(pred, 1)
```

```
##    1
## 1.6
```

Now, let's say we want to know the expected number of asthmatic attacks per year for those with and without recurrent respiratory infection for each 12-mark increase in GHQ-12 score.

```
new_data = data.frame(res_inf = rep(c("yes", "no"), each = 4),
                      ghq12 = rep(c(0, 12, 24, 36), 2))
new_data$attack_pred = round(predict(pois_attack_final, new_data,
                             type = "response"), 1)
new_data
```

```
##    res_inf ghq12 attack_pred
## 1      yes     0         1.1
## 2      yes    12         2.0
## 3      yes    24         3.6
## 4      yes    36         6.6
## 5       no     0         0.7
## 6       no    12         1.3
## 7       no    24         2.4
## 8       no    36         4.3
```

10.5   Poisson Regression for Rate

10.5.1   About Poisson regression for rate

At times, the count is proportional to a denominator. For example, given the same number of deaths, the death rate in a small population will be higher than the rate in a large population. If we were to compare the number of deaths between the populations, it would not make a fair comparison. Thus, we may consider adding denominators in the Poisson regression modeling in form of offsets. This denominator could also be the unit time of exposure, for example person-years of cigarette smoking.

As mentioned before, counts can be proportional specific denominators, giving rise to rates. We may add the denominators in the Poisson regression modeling as offsets. Again, these denominators could be stratum size or unit time of exposure. Multiple Poisson regression for rate is specified by adding the offset in the form of the natural log of the denominator t. This is given as,

$$ln(\hat{y}) = ln(t) + b_0 + b_1x_1 + b_2x_2 + ... + b_px_p$$

10.5.2   Dataset

The data on the number of lung cancer cases among doctors, cigarettes per day, years of smoking and the respective person-years at risk of lung cancer are given in smoke.csv. The person-years variable serves as the offset for our analysis. The original data came from Doll (1971), which were analyzed in the context of Poisson regression by Frome (1983) and Fleiss et al. (2003). The dataset contains four variables:

1. *smoke_yrs*: Years of smoking (categorical) {15-19, 204-24, 25-29, 30-34, 35-39, 40-44, 45-49, 50-54, 55-59}.
2. *cigar_day*: Cigarettes per day (numerical).
3. *person_yrs*: Person-years at risk of lung cancer (numerical).
4. *case*: Number of lung cancer cases (count).

The dataset is loaded as follows,

```
smoke = read.csv("data/smoke.csv")
```

Then, we look at its data structure,

```
str(smoke)
```

```
## 'data.frame':    63 obs. of  4 variables:
```

```
##  $ smoke_yrs : chr  "15-19" "20-24" "25-29" "30-34" ...
##  $ cigar_day : num  0 0 0 0 0 0 0 0 0 5.2 ...
##  $ person_yrs: int  10366 8162 5969 4496 3512 2201 1421 1121 826 3121 ...
##  $ case      : int  1 0 0 0 0 0 0 0 2 0 ...
```

10.5.3   Data exploration

For descriptive statistics, we use `epidisplay::codebook` as before.

```
epiDisplay::codebook(smoke)
```

```
##
##
##
## smoke_yrs    :
## A character vector
##
##  =================
## cigar_day    :
##  obs. mean    median   s.d.     min.    max.
##  63   17.271 15.9     12.913  0       40.8
##
##  =================
## person_yrs   :
##  obs. mean       median   s.d.       min.    max.
##  63   2426.444 1826     2030.143  104      10366
##
##  =================
## case     :
##  obs. mean    median   s.d.     min.    max.
##  63   2.698  1        3.329   0       12
##
##  =================
```

In addition, we are also interested to look at the observed rates,

```
smoke %>% mutate(rate = round(case/person_yrs, 4))
```

```
##     smoke_yrs cigar_day person_yrs case   rate
## 1     15-19       0.0      10366    1 0.0001
## 2     20-24       0.0       8162    0 0.0000
## 3     25-29       0.0       5969    0 0.0000
## 4     30-34       0.0       4496    0 0.0000
## 5     35-39       0.0       3512    0 0.0000
```

```
## 6     40-44     0.0     2201     0 0.0000
## 7     45-49     0.0     1421     0 0.0000
## 8     50-54     0.0     1121     0 0.0000
## 9     55-59     0.0      826     2 0.0024
## 10    15-19     5.2     3121     0 0.0000
## 11    20-24     5.2     2937     0 0.0000
## 12    25-29     5.2     2288     0 0.0000
## 13    30-34     5.2     2015     0 0.0000
## 14    35-39     5.2     1648     1 0.0006
## 15    40-44     5.2     1310     2 0.0015
## 16    45-49     5.2      927     0 0.0000
## 17    50-54     5.2      710     3 0.0042
## 18    55-59     5.2      606     0 0.0000
## 19    15-19    11.2     3577     0 0.0000
## 20    20-24    11.2     3286     1 0.0003
## 21    25-29    11.2     2546     1 0.0004
## 22    30-34    11.2     2219     2 0.0009
## 23    35-39    11.2     1826     0 0.0000
## 24    40-44    11.2     1386     1 0.0007
## 25    45-49    11.2      988     2 0.0020
## 26    50-54    11.2      684     4 0.0058
## 27    55-59    11.2      449     3 0.0067
## 28    15-19    15.9     4317     0 0.0000
## 29    20-24    15.9     4214     0 0.0000
## 30    25-29    15.9     3185     0 0.0000
## 31    30-34    15.9     2560     4 0.0016
## 32    35-39    15.9     1893     0 0.0000
## 33    40-44    15.9     1334     2 0.0015
## 34    45-49    15.9      849     2 0.0024
## 35    50-54    15.9      470     2 0.0043
## 36    55-59    15.9      280     5 0.0179
## 37    15-19    20.4     5683     0 0.0000
## 38    20-24    20.4     6385     1 0.0002
## 39    25-29    20.4     5483     1 0.0002
## 40    30-34    20.4     4687     6 0.0013
## 41    35-39    20.4     3646     5 0.0014
## 42    40-44    20.4     2411    12 0.0050
## 43    45-49    20.4     1567     9 0.0057
## 44    50-54    20.4      857     7 0.0082
## 45    55-59    20.4      416     7 0.0168
## 46    15-19    27.4     3042     0 0.0000
## 47    20-24    27.4     4050     1 0.0002
## 48    25-29    27.4     4290     4 0.0009
## 49    30-34    27.4     4268     9 0.0021
## 50    35-39    27.4     3529     9 0.0026
```

```
## 51    40-44    27.4    2424   11 0.0045
## 52    45-49    27.4    1409   10 0.0071
## 53    50-54    27.4     663    5 0.0075
## 54    55-59    27.4     284    3 0.0106
## 55    15-19    40.8     670    0 0.0000
## 56    20-24    40.8    1166    0 0.0000
## 57    25-29    40.8    1482    0 0.0000
## 58    30-34    40.8    1580    4 0.0025
## 59    35-39    40.8    1336    6 0.0045
## 60    40-44    40.8     924   10 0.0108
## 61    45-49    40.8     556    7 0.0126
## 62    50-54    40.8     255    4 0.0157
## 63    55-59    40.8     104    1 0.0096
```

10.5.4 Univariable analysis

For the univariable analysis, we fit univariable Poisson regression models for cigarettes per day (cigar_day), and years of smoking (smoke_yrs) variables. Offset or denominator is included as offset = log(person_yrs) in the glm option.

```
# cigar_day
pois_case1 = glm(case ~ cigar_day, data = smoke, family = "poisson",
                 offset = log(person_yrs))
summary(pois_case1)
```

```
##
## Call:
## glm(formula = case ~ cigar_day, family = "poisson", data = smoke,
##     offset = log(person_yrs))
##
## Deviance Residuals:
##     Min      1Q   Median      3Q      Max
## -3.8684  -1.6542  -0.5111  1.8415   4.8937
##
## Coefficients:
##             Estimate Std. Error z value Pr(>|z|)
## (Intercept) -8.159268   0.175063  -46.61   <2e-16 ***
## cigar_day    0.070359   0.006468   10.88   <2e-16 ***
## ---
## Signif. codes:  0 '***' 0.001 '**' 0.01 '*' 0.05 '.' 0.1 ' ' 1
##
## (Dispersion parameter for poisson family taken to be 1)
##
##     Null deviance: 445.10  on 62  degrees of freedom
```

```
## Residual deviance: 324.71  on 61  degrees of freedom
## AIC: 448.55
##
## Number of Fisher Scoring iterations: 6
```

```
# smoke_yrs
pois_case2 = glm(case ~ smoke_yrs, data = smoke, family = "poisson",
                 offset = log(person_yrs))
summary(pois_case2)
```

```
##
## Call:
## glm(formula = case ~ smoke_yrs, family = "poisson", data = smoke,
##     offset = log(person_yrs))
##
## Deviance Residuals:
##     Min      1Q   Median      3Q      Max
## -3.7351  -1.1923  -0.3531   0.9332   3.2279
##
## Coefficients:
##                  Estimate Std. Error z value Pr(>|z|)
## (Intercept)       -10.335      1.000 -10.335  < 2e-16 ***
## smoke_yrs20-24      1.117      1.155   0.968 0.333149
## smoke_yrs25-29      1.990      1.080   1.842 0.065423 .
## smoke_yrs30-34      3.563      1.020   3.493 0.000477 ***
## smoke_yrs35-39      3.615      1.024   3.532 0.000412 ***
## smoke_yrs40-44      4.580      1.013   4.521 6.15e-06 ***
## smoke_yrs45-49      4.785      1.016   4.707 2.52e-06 ***
## smoke_yrs50-54      5.085      1.020   4.987 6.14e-07 ***
## smoke_yrs55-59      5.384      1.024   5.261 1.44e-07 ***
## ---
## Signif. codes:  0 '***' 0.001 '**' 0.01 '*' 0.05 '.' 0.1 ' ' 1
##
## (Dispersion parameter for poisson family taken to be 1)
##
##     Null deviance: 445.10  on 62  degrees of freedom
## Residual deviance: 170.17  on 54  degrees of freedom
## AIC: 308.01
##
## Number of Fisher Scoring iterations: 5
```

From the outputs, all variables including the dummy variables are important with p-values $< .25$.

10.5.5   Multivariable analysis

For the multivariable analysis, we included `cigar_day` and `smoke_yrs` as predictors of case.

```
pois_case = glm(case ~ cigar_day + smoke_yrs, data = smoke,
                family = "poisson", offset = log(person_yrs))
summary(pois_case)
```

```
##
## Call:
## glm(formula = case ~ cigar_day + smoke_yrs, family = "poisson",
##     data = smoke, offset = log(person_yrs))
##
## Deviance Residuals:
##     Min       1Q    Median        3Q       Max
## -2.1066  -0.9404   -0.3337    0.4366    1.7439
##
## Coefficients:
##                   Estimate Std. Error z value Pr(>|z|)
## (Intercept)     -11.317162   1.007492 -11.233  < 2e-16 ***
## cigar_day         0.064361   0.006401  10.054  < 2e-16 ***
## smoke_yrs20-24    0.962417   1.154694   0.833  0.40457
## smoke_yrs25-29    1.710894   1.080420   1.584  0.11330
## smoke_yrs30-34    3.207676   1.020378   3.144  0.00167 **
## smoke_yrs35-39    3.242776   1.024187   3.166  0.00154 **
## smoke_yrs40-44    4.208361   1.013726   4.151 3.30e-05 ***
## smoke_yrs45-49    4.448972   1.017054   4.374 1.22e-05 ***
## smoke_yrs50-54    4.893674   1.019945   4.798 1.60e-06 ***
## smoke_yrs55-59    5.372600   1.023404   5.250 1.52e-07 ***
## ---
## Signif. codes:  0 '***' 0.001 '**' 0.01 '*' 0.05 '.' 0.1 ' ' 1
##
## (Dispersion parameter for poisson family taken to be 1)
##
##     Null deviance: 445.099  on 62  degrees of freedom
## Residual deviance:  68.015  on 53  degrees of freedom
## AIC: 207.86
##
## Number of Fisher Scoring iterations: 5
```

From the output, both variables are significant predictors of the rate of lung cancer cases, although we noted the *p*-values are not significant for `smoke_yrs20-24` and `smoke_yrs25-29` dummy variables. This model serves as our **preliminary model**.

10.5.6 Interaction

Now, we include a two-way interaction term between cigar_day and smoke_yrs. From the output, although we noted that the interaction terms are not significant, the standard errors for cigar_day and the interaction terms are extremely large. This might point to a numerical issue with the model (Hosmer et al., 2013). So, we may drop the interaction term from our model.

```
pois_casex = glm(case ~ cigar_day * smoke_yrs, data = smoke,
                 family = "poisson", offset = log(person_yrs))


## Warning: glm.fit: fitted rates numerically 0 occurred


summary(pois_casex)


##
## Call:
## glm(formula = case ~ cigar_day * smoke_yrs, family = "poisson",
##     data = smoke, offset = log(person_yrs))
##
## Deviance Residuals:
##     Min      1Q  Median      3Q     Max
## -2.3232  -0.8816  -0.1886  0.4965  1.6851
##
## Coefficients:
##                           Estimate Std. Error z value Pr(>|z|)
## (Intercept)                -9.2463     1.0000  -9.246  < 2e-16 ***
## cigar_day                  -2.8137   319.6350  -0.009 0.992976
## smoke_yrs20-24             -0.7514     1.5114  -0.497 0.619084
## smoke_yrs25-29             -0.2539     1.3518  -0.188 0.851030
## smoke_yrs30-34              1.2493     1.1032   1.132 0.257489
## smoke_yrs35-39              0.5856     1.1660   0.502 0.615498
## smoke_yrs40-44              1.9706     1.0790   1.826 0.067800 .
## smoke_yrs45-49              2.1070     1.0982   1.919 0.055044 .
## smoke_yrs50-54              3.0710     1.0761   2.854 0.004318 **
## smoke_yrs55-59              3.5704     1.0706   3.335 0.000853 ***
## cigar_day:smoke_yrs20-24    2.8609   319.6351   0.009 0.992859
## cigar_day:smoke_yrs25-29    2.8736   319.6351   0.009 0.992827
## cigar_day:smoke_yrs30-34    2.8736   319.6350   0.009 0.992827
## cigar_day:smoke_yrs35-39    2.8997   319.6350   0.009 0.992762
## cigar_day:smoke_yrs40-44    2.8845   319.6350   0.009 0.992800
## cigar_day:smoke_yrs45-49    2.8886   319.6350   0.009 0.992790
## cigar_day:smoke_yrs50-54    2.8669   319.6350   0.009 0.992844
## cigar_day:smoke_yrs55-59    2.8641   319.6350   0.009 0.992851
```

```
## ---
## Signif. codes:  0 '***' 0.001 '**' 0.01 '*' 0.05 '.' 0.1 ' ' 1
##
## (Dispersion parameter for poisson family taken to be 1)
##
##     Null deviance: 445.099  on 62  degrees of freedom
## Residual deviance:  60.597  on 45  degrees of freedom
## AIC: 216.44
##
## Number of Fisher Scoring iterations: 18
```

10.5.7   Model fit assessment

Again, we assess the model fit by chi-square goodness-of-fit test, model-to-model AIC comparison and scaled Pearson chi-square statistic and standardized residuals.

```
# Chi-square goodness-of-fit
epiDisplay::poisgof(pois_case)
```

```
## $results
## [1] "Goodness-of-fit test for Poisson assumption"
##
## $chisq
## [1] 68.01514
##
## $df
## [1] 53
##
## $p.value
## [1] 0.0802866
```

The *p*-value of chi-square goodness-of-fit is more than 0.05, which indicates the model has good fit.

```
# Model-to-model AIC comparison
AIC(pois_case1, pois_case2, pois_case)
```

```
##             df      AIC
## pois_case1   2 448.5549
## pois_case2   9 308.0129
## pois_case   10 207.8574
```

The comparison by AIC clearly shows that the multivariable model pois_case is the best model as it has the lowest AIC value.

```
# Scaled Pearson chi-square statistic using quasipoisson
qpois_case_summ = summary(glm(case ~ cigar_day + smoke_yrs, data = smoke,
                               family = "quasipoisson",
                               offset = log(person_yrs)))
qpois_case_summ$dispersion
```

```
## [1] 1.072516
```

The value of dispersion, i.e. the scaled Pearson chi-square statistic, is close to 1. This again indicates that the model has good fit.

```
# Standardized residuals
std_res = rstandard(pois_case)
std_res[abs(std_res) > 1.96]
```

```
##          6          8         18
## -1.995530 -2.025055 -2.253832
```

```
index = names(std_res[abs(std_res) > 1.96])
# points of discrepancies
cbind(smoke[index,], case_pred = pois_case$fitted[index]) %>%
  mutate(rate = round(case/person_yrs, 4),
         rate_pred = round(case_pred/person_yrs, 4))
```

```
##    smoke_yrs cigar_day person_yrs case case_pred rate rate_pred
## 6      40-44       0.0       2201    0  1.800143    0    0.0008
## 8      50-54       0.0       1121    0  1.819366    0    0.0016
## 18     55-59       5.2        606    0  2.218868    0    0.0037
```

Lastly, we noted only a few observations (number 6, 8 and 18) have discrepancies between the observed and predicted cases. This shows how well the fitted Poisson regression model for rate explains the data at hand.

10.5.8 Presentation and interpretation

Now, we decide on the final model,

```
pois_case_final = pois_case
```

and use `tbl_regression()` to come up with a table for the results. Again, for interpretation, we exponentiate the coefficients to obtain the incidence rate ratio, *IRR*.

```
tbl_regression(pois_case_final, exponentiate = TRUE)
```

Characteristic	IRR[1]	95% CI[1]	p-value
cigar_day	1.07	1.05, 1.08	< 0.001
smoke_yrs			
15-19	—	—	
20-24	2.62	0.34, 52.9	0.4
25-29	5.53	0.94, 105	0.11
30-34	24.7	5.23, 442	0.002
35-39	25.6	5.35, 459	0.002
40-44	67.2	14.6, 1,195	< 0.001
45-49	85.5	18.3, 1,525	< 0.001
50-54	133	28.3, 2,385	< 0.001
55-59	215	45.1, 3,862	< 0.001

[1]IRR = Incidence Rate Ratio, CI = Confidence Interval

From this table, we interpret the IRR values as follows:

- Taking an additional cigarette per day increases the risk of having lung cancer by 1.07 (95% CI: 1.05, 1.08), while controlling for the other variables.
- Those who had been smoking for between 30 to 34 years are at higher risk of having lung cancer with an IRR of 24.7 (95% CI: 5.23, 442), while controlling for the other variables.

We leave the rest of the IRRs for you to interpret. But take note that the IRRs for years of smoking (smoke_yrs) between 30-34 to 55-59 categories are quite large with wide 95% CIs, although this does not seem to be a problem since the standard errors are reasonable for the estimated coefficients (look again at summary(pois_case)). The 95% CIs for 20-24 and 25-29 include 1 (which means no risk) with risks ranging from lower risk (IRR < 1) to higher risk (IRR > 1). This is expected because the p-values for these two categories are not significant.

Then, we view and save the output in the spreadsheet format for later use. We use tidy(),

```
tib_pois_case = tidy(pois_case_final, exponentiate = TRUE,
                     conf.int = TRUE)
tib_pois_case
```

```
## # A tibble: 10 x 7
##    term            estimate std.error statistic  p.value  conf.low conf.high
##    <chr>              <dbl>     <dbl>     <dbl>    <dbl>     <dbl>     <dbl>
## 1 (Intercept)    0.0000122      1.01     -11.2  2.81e-29   6.89e-7   5.49e-5
```

```
##  2 cigar_day         1.07      0.00640   10.1  8.79e-24    1.05e+0   1.08e+0
##  3 smoke_yrs20-24    2.62      1.15            0.833 4.05e- 1   3.35e-1   5.29e+1
##  4 smoke_yrs25-29    5.53      1.08            1.58  1.13e- 1   9.44e-1   1.05e+2
##  5 smoke_yrs30-34   24.7       1.02            3.14  1.67e- 3   5.23e+0   4.42e+2
##  6 smoke_yrs35-39   25.6       1.02            3.17  1.54e- 3   5.35e+0   4.59e+2
##  7 smoke_yrs40-44   67.2       1.01            4.15  3.30e- 5   1.46e+1   1.19e+3
##  8 smoke_yrs45-49   85.5       1.02            4.37  1.22e- 5   1.83e+1   1.52e+3
##  9 smoke_yrs50-54  133.        1.02            4.80  1.60e- 6   2.83e+1   2.38e+3
## 10 smoke_yrs55-59  215.        1.02            5.25  1.52e- 7   4.51e+1   3.86e+3
```

and export it to a .csv file,

```
write.csv(tib_pois_case, "tib_pois_case.csv")
```

Now, we present the model equation, which unfortunately this time quite a lengthy one. We display the coefficients,

```
round(summary(pois_case_final)$coefficients, 2)
```

```
##                  Estimate Std. Error z value Pr(>|z|)
## (Intercept)       -11.32       1.01  -11.23     0.00
## cigar_day           0.06       0.01   10.05     0.00
## smoke_yrs20-24      0.96       1.15    0.83     0.40
## smoke_yrs25-29      1.71       1.08    1.58     0.11
## smoke_yrs30-34      3.21       1.02    3.14     0.00
## smoke_yrs35-39      3.24       1.02    3.17     0.00
## smoke_yrs40-44      4.21       1.01    4.15     0.00
## smoke_yrs45-49      4.45       1.02    4.37     0.00
## smoke_yrs50-54      4.89       1.02    4.80     0.00
## smoke_yrs55-59      5.37       1.02    5.25     0.00
```

and put the values in the equation. Remember to include the offset in the equation.

$$
\begin{aligned}
ln(case) = {} & ln(person\_yrs) - 11.32 + 0.06 \times cigar\_day \\
& + 0.96 \times smoke\_yrs(20-24) + 1.71 \times smoke\_yrs(25-29) \\
& + 3.21 \times smoke\_yrs(30-34) + 3.24 \times smoke\_yrs(35-39) \\
& + 4.21 \times smoke\_yrs(40-44) + 4.45 \times smoke\_yrs(45-49) \\
& + 4.89 \times smoke\_yrs(50-54) + 5.37 \times smoke\_yrs(55-59)
\end{aligned}
$$

10.6   Quasi-Poisson Regression for Overdispersed Data

We utilized `family = "quasipoisson"` option in the `glm` specification before just to easily obtain the scaled Pearson chi-square statistic without knowing what it is. So, what is a quasi-Poisson regression? For a typical Poisson regression analysis, we rely on maximum likelihood estimation method. It assumes that the mean (of the count) and its variance are equal, or variance divided by mean equals 1. For that reason, we expect that scaled Pearson chi-square statistic to be close to 1 so as to indicate good fit of the Poisson regression model.

So what if this assumption of "mean equals variance" is violated? Whenever the variance is larger than the mean for that model, we call this issue *overdispersion*. In particular, it will affect a Poisson regression model by underestimating the standard errors of the coefficients. So, we may have narrower confidence intervals and smaller p-values (i.e. more likely to have false positive results) than what we could have obtained. In handling the overdispersion issue, one may use a negative binomial regression, which we do not cover in this book. A more flexible option is by using quasi-Poisson regression that relies on quasi-likelihood estimation method (Fleiss et al., 2003).

To demonstrate a quasi-Poisson regression is not difficult because we already did that before when we wanted to obtain scaled Pearson chi-square statistic before in the previous sections. As an example, we repeat the same using the model for count. We fit the standard Poisson regression model,

```
pois_attack_all1 = glm(attack ~ ., data = asthma, family = "poisson")
```

Then we fit the same model using quasi-Poisson regression,

```
qpois_attack_all1 = glm(attack ~ ., data = asthma,
                        family = "quasipoisson")
```

Now, pay attention to the standard errors and confidence intervals of each models. Can you spot the differences between the two? (Hints: `std.error`, `p.value`, `conf.low` and `conf.high` columns).

```
# Poisson
tidy(pois_attack_all1, conf.int = TRUE)
```

```
## # A tibble: 4 x 7
##    term        estimate std.error statistic  p.value conf.low conf.high
##    <chr>          <dbl>     <dbl>     <dbl>    <dbl>    <dbl>     <dbl>
```

```
## 1 (Intercept)  -0.315   0.183     -1.72  8.57e- 2  -0.685   0.0347
## 2 gendermale   -0.0419  0.122     -0.342 7.32e- 1  -0.285   0.196
## 3 res_infyes    0.426   0.153      2.79  5.28e- 3   0.133   0.733
## 4 ghq12         0.0495  0.00788    6.28  3.29e-10   0.0342  0.0651


# quasi-Poisson
tidy(qpois_attack_all1, conf.int = TRUE)


## # A tibble: 4 x 7
##    term         estimate std.error statistic    p.value conf.low conf.high
##    <chr>           <dbl>     <dbl>     <dbl>      <dbl>    <dbl>     <dbl>
## 1 (Intercept)   -0.315     0.189     -1.67  0.0979      -0.697   0.0449
## 2 gendermale    -0.0419    0.126     -0.332 0.740       -0.292   0.203
## 3 res_infyes     0.426     0.157      2.71  0.00779      0.124   0.742
## 4 ghq12          0.0495    0.00812    6.10  0.0000000143 0.0337  0.0656
```

Note that there are no changes to the coefficients between the standard Poisson regression and the quasi-Poisson regression. We also interpret the quasi-Poisson regression model output in the same way to that of the standard Poisson regression model output.

10.7 Summary

In this chapter, we went through the basics about Poisson regression for count and rate data. We performed the analysis for each and learned how to assess the model fit for the regression models. We learned how to nicely present and interpret the results. In addition, we also learned how to utilize the model for prediction.To understand more about the concep, analysis workflow and interpretation of count data analysis including Poisson regression, we recommend texts from the Epidemiology: Study Design and Data Analysis book (Woodward, 2013) and Regression Models for Categorical Dependent Variables Using Stata book (Long et al., 2006).

11

Survival Analysis: Kaplan–Meier and Cox Proportional Hazard (PH) Regression

11.1 Objectives

At the end of the chapter, the readers will be

- to understand the basic concept of non-parametric survival analysis such as the Kaplan–Meier estimates and the semi-parametric survival analysis such the Cox proportional hazard (PH) regression.
- to perform the Kaplan–Meier analysis
- to test the hypothesis of the survival distributions for two samples.
- to perform the simple (univariable) Cox PH regression analysis
- to perform the multiple (multivariable) Cox PH regression analysis

11.2 Introduction

Regression concerns the relationship between a response variable and one or more exploratory variables. The independent variables are also called covariates. Some common regression analysis in health and medicine is linear regression, logistic regression, Poisson regression and Cox proportional hazards regression. Linear regression falls under the general linear model while the other three regression models fall under the generalized linear regression.

Survival analysis is also known as duration analysis or time-to-event analysis. This analysis is useful in follow up studies where participants or patients are followed-up until they develop the event of interest. Examples of such studies include the retrospective cohort or prospective cohort studies.

Sometime people confuse and wrongly think that the survival analysis is only applicable to the study of survival (where the event of interest is either alive or death condition). It is not. Any study that involves both the duration of follow up (in days or weeks or months) and the event of interest can be considered as suitable for survival analysis. So, survival or duration analysis is performed on data that has duration until an event occurs.

In health and medicine studies, this event can be of interest, for example:

- relapse after treatment
- death after diagnosis
- recurrence of disease
- treatment success

And for variable time, it can be in any time form such as days, weeks, years or event minutes. If we combine them together (with the event of interest) then it can become:

- months to relapse
- years from diagnosis to death
- weeks before recurrence
- days taken from the start of treatment to treatment success

11.3   Types of Survival Analysis

There are three main types of survival analysis:

- the non-parametric survival analysis for example Kaplan–Meier estimates.
- the semi-parametric survival analysis for example Cox proportional hazards (PH) regression.
- the parametric survival analysis for example Weibull parametric survival analysis.

In medical literature, we usually perform the non-parametric analysis for example the Kaplan–Meier estimates at the beginning of the analysis to understand the trend of survival probabilities. Following that, we perform simple (univariable) or multiple (multivariable) Cox proportional hazard (PH) regression model. If we are sure with the distribution of the risk and aim to estimate the survival time, then we can perform parametric survival analysis.

11.4   Prepare Environment for Analysis

11.4.1   RStudio project

We recommend your start a new analysis project by creating a new RStudio project. To do this:

1. Go to File
2. Click New Project
3. Choose New Directory or Existing Directory.

This directory actually a folder that should contain the R codes, the dataset and the outputs from the analysis. To organize further, we would create a folder and name it as data in the directory. And we will copy the dataset stroke_data.csv in the data folder.

11.4.2 Packages

Next, we will load the necessary packages. We will use these packages:

- **gtsummary**: a package that give us a nice formatted tables of statistics
- **tidyverse**: a package for data wrangling and making plots
- **lubridate** : a package to manipulate dates
- **survival**: a package to run survival analysis.
- **survminer**: a package to plot survival objects
- **broom**: a package to make prettier outputs
- **here** : a package to manage location fo files

In addition to **survival** package, there are other packages that can perform survival analysis. The details of the package is available here https://cran.r-project.org/web/views/Survival.html.

Now, we will load the packages:

```
library(here)
```

```
## here() starts at C:/Users/drkim/Downloads/multivar_data_analysis/multivar_data_analysis
```

```
library(tidyverse)
```

```
## -- Attaching core tidyverse packages ------------------------ tidyverse 2.0.0 -
-
## v dplyr     1.1.1     v readr     2.1.4
## v forcats   1.0.0     v stringr   1.5.0
## v ggplot2   3.4.2     v tibble    3.2.1
## v lubridate 1.9.2     v tidyr     1.3.0
## v purrr     1.0.1
## 
##          --          Conflicts          -----------------------------------------
tidyverse_conflicts() --
## x dplyr::filter() masks stats::filter()
## x dplyr::lag()     masks stats::lag()
```

```
##    i    Use    the    conflicted    package    (<http://conflicted.r-
lib.org/>) to force all conflicts to become errors
```

```
library(lubridate)
library(survival)
library(survminer)
```

```
## Loading required package: ggpubr
##
## Attaching package: 'survminer'
##
## The following object is masked from 'package:survival':
##
##    myeloma
```

```
library(broom)
library(gtsummary)
```

Remember, check if all packages are available in your R library. If not, you will receive an error message stating that the package is not available. To install the package, use the `install.packages()` function. It will download and install the packages to your R libraries. Once the packages are installed, load the packages again using the `library()` function.

11.5   Data

The tutorial uses a dataset named `stroke_data.csv`. This is comma-separated value dataset. Now let us load the data

```
stroke <- read_csv(here('data', 'stroke_data.csv'))
```

```
## Rows: 213 Columns: 12
## -- Column specification ----------------------------------------------
---
## Delimiter: ","
## chr (7): doa, dod, status, sex, dm, stroke_type, referral_from
## dbl (5): gcs, sbp, dbp, wbc, time2
##
## i Use `spec()` to retrieve the full column specification for this data.
## i Specify the column types or set `show_col_types = FALSE` to quiet this message.
```

And take a peek at our data to check

- number of observations (n=213)
- name of variables (12 variables)
- type of variables (character and double)

```
glimpse(stroke)
```

```
## Rows: 213
## Columns: 12
## $ doa          <chr> "17/2/2011", "20/3/2011", "9/4/2011", "12/4/2011", "12/4~
## $ dod          <chr> "18/2/2011", "21/3/2011", "10/4/2011", "13/4/2011", "13/~
## $ status       <chr> "alive", "alive", "dead", "dead", "alive", "dead", "aliv~
## $ sex          <chr> "male", "male", "female", "male", "female", "female", "m~
## $ dm           <chr> "no", "no", "no", "no", "yes", "no", "no", "yes", "yes",~
## $ gcs          <dbl> 15, 15, 11, 3, 15, 3, 11, 15, 6, 15, 15, 4, 4, 10, 12, 1~
## $ sbp          <dbl> 151, 196, 126, 170, 103, 91, 171, 106, 170, 123, 144, 23~
## $ dbp          <dbl> 73, 123, 78, 103, 62, 55, 80, 67, 90, 83, 89, 120, 120, ~
## $ wbc          <dbl> 12.5, 8.1, 15.3, 13.9, 14.7, 14.2, 8.7, 5.5, 10.5, 7.2, ~
## $ time2        <dbl> 1, 1, 1, 1, 1, 1, 1, 1, 1, 1, 1, 1, 1, 1, 1, 1, 1, 1, 1,~
## $ stroke_type  <chr> "IS", "IS", "HS", "IS", "IS", "HS", "IS", "IS", "HS", "I~
## $ referral_from <chr> "non-hospital", "non-hospital", "hospital", "hospital", ~
```

These data come from patients who were admitted at a tertiary hospital due to acute stroke. They were treated in the ward and the status (dead or alive) were recorded. The variables are:

- doa : date of admission
- dod : date of discharge
- status : event at discharge (alive or dead)
- sex : male or female
- dm : diabetes (yes or no)
- gcs : Glasgow Coma Scale (value from 3 to 15)
- sbp : Systolic blood pressure (mmHg)
- dbp : Diastolic blood pressure (mmHg)
- wbc : Total white cell count
- time2 : days in ward
- stroke_type : stroke type (Ischemic stroke or Hemorrhagic stroke)
- referral_from : patient was referred from a hospital or not from a hospital

The outcome of interest is time from admission to death. The time variable is `time2` (in days) and the event variable is `status`. The event of interest is `dead`. We also note that variables dates and other categorical variables are in character format. The rest are in numerical format.

11.6 Explore Data

We will convert the variable doa and variable doa to a more valid format (date format):

```
stroke <-
  stroke %>%
  mutate(doa = dmy(doa),
         dod = dmy(dod))
```

We will perform a quick preliminary analysis. First, by looking at the summary statistics:

```
summary(stroke)
```

```
##       doa                  dod                 status
##   Min.   :2011-01-01   Min.   :2011-01-05   Length:213
##   1st Qu.:2011-06-06   1st Qu.:2011-06-09   Class :character
##   Median :2011-10-31   Median :2011-11-02   Mode  :character
##   Mean   :2011-10-16   Mean   :2011-10-23
##   3rd Qu.:2012-03-12   3rd Qu.:2012-03-18
##   Max.   :2012-06-23   Max.   :2012-06-27
##       sex                  dm                  gcs                sbp
##   Length:213           Length:213          Min.   : 3.00    Min.   : 75.0
##   Class :character     Class :character    1st Qu.:10.00    1st Qu.:142.0
##   Mode  :character     Mode  :character    Median :15.00    Median :160.0
##                                            Mean   :12.52    Mean   :162.8
##                                            3rd Qu.:15.00    3rd Qu.:186.0
##                                            Max.   :15.00    Max.   :290.0
##       dbp                wbc               time2           stroke_type
##   Min.   : 42.00   Min.   : 4.2     Min.   : 1.000    Length:213
##   1st Qu.: 79.00   1st Qu.: 7.5     1st Qu.: 3.000    Class :character
##   Median : 90.00   Median : 9.9     Median : 4.000    Mode  :character
##   Mean   : 91.53   Mean   :10.4     Mean   : 6.474
##   3rd Qu.:103.00   3rd Qu.:12.5     3rd Qu.: 7.000
##   Max.   :160.00   Max.   :27.0     Max.   :43.000
```

```
##   referral_from
##   Length:213
##   Class :character
##   Mode  :character
##
##
##
```

The `tbl_summary()` function from **gtsummary** package can produce nice tables. For example, the overall characteristics of patients can be obtained by:

```
stroke %>%
  tbl_summary() %>%
  as_gt()
```

Characteristic	N = 213[1]
doa	2011-01-01 to 2012-06-23
dod	2011-01-05 to 2012-06-27
status	
alive	165 (77%)
dead	48 (23%)
sex	
female	122 (57%)
male	91 (43%)
dm	72 (34%)
gcs	15.0 (10.0, 15.0)
sbp	160 (142, 186)
dbp	90 (79, 103)
wbc	9.9 (7.5, 12.5)
time2	4 (3, 7)
stroke_type	
HS	69 (32%)
IS	144 (68%)
referral_from	
hospital	80 (38%)
non-hospital	133 (62%)

[1]Range; n (%); Median (IQR)

To obtain the patients characteristics based on status:

```
stroke %>%
  tbl_summary(by = status) %>%
  as_gt()
```

Characteristic	alive, N = 165[1]	dead, N = 48[1]
doa	2011-01-03 to 2012-06-22	2011-01-01 to 2012-06-23
dod	2011-01-06 to 2012-06-27	2011-01-05 to 2012-06-26
sex		
female	87 (53%)	35 (73%)
male	78 (47%)	13 (27%)
dm	59 (36%)	13 (27%)
gcs	15.0 (14.0, 15.0)	8.5 (5.0, 11.2)
sbp	160 (143, 186)	162 (137, 192)
dbp	90 (79, 102)	90 (80, 109)
wbc	9.0 (7.2, 11.6)	11.4 (10.0, 14.5)
time2	4 (3, 6)	5 (2, 12)
stroke_type		
HS	38 (23%)	31 (65%)
IS	127 (77%)	17 (35%)
referral_from		
hospital	51 (31%)	29 (60%)
non-hospital	114 (69%)	19 (40%)

[1]Range; n (%); Median (IQR)

To obtain the patients characteristics based on stroke types:

```
stroke %>%
  tbl_summary(by = stroke_type) %>%
  as_gt()
```

Characteristic	HS, N = 69[1]	IS, N = 144[1]
doa	2011-01-06 to 2012-06-23	2011-01-01 to 2012-06-16
dod	2011-01-22 to 2012-06-26	2011-01-05 to 2012-06-27
status		
alive	38 (55%)	127 (88%)
dead	31 (45%)	17 (12%)
sex		
female	43 (62%)	79 (55%)

male	26 (38%)	65 (45%)
dm	19 (28%)	53 (37%)
gcs	11.0 (6.0, 14.0)	15.0 (13.8, 15.0)
sbp	152 (139, 187)	161 (143, 186)
dbp	90 (80, 102)	91 (79, 103)
wbc	11.4 (9.4, 14.9)	8.8 (7.2, 11.1)
time2	6 (4, 15)	4 (3, 5)
referral_from		
hospital	46 (67%)	34 (24%)
non-hospital	23 (33%)	110 (76%)

[1]Range; n (%); Median (IQR)

11.7 Kaplan–Meier Survival Estimates

Kaplan–Meier survival estimates is the non-parametric survival estimates. It provides the survival probability estimates at different time. Using survfit(), we can estimate the survival probability based on Kaplan–Meier (KM).

Let's estimate the survival probabilities for

- overall
- stroke types

The survival probabilities for all patients:

```
KM <- survfit(Surv(time = time2,
                   event = status == "dead" ) ~ 1,
              data = stroke)
summary(KM)
```

```
## Call: survfit(formula = Surv(time = time2, event = status == "dead") ~
##      1, data = stroke)
##
##  time n.risk n.event survival std.err lower 95% CI upper 95% CI
##     1    213       9    0.958  0.0138       0.9311        0.985
##     2    190       4    0.938  0.0168       0.9053        0.971
##     3    166       4    0.915  0.0198       0.8770        0.955
##     4    130       4    0.887  0.0237       0.8416        0.934
##     5     90       5    0.838  0.0310       0.7790        0.901
##     6     65       3    0.799  0.0367       0.7301        0.874
##     7     56       4    0.742  0.0438       0.6608        0.833
##     9     42       1    0.724  0.0462       0.6391        0.821
```

```
##     10     37     1     0.705   0.0489        0.6150        0.807
##     12     33     4     0.619   0.0587        0.5142        0.746
##     14     24     2     0.568   0.0642        0.4548        0.708
##     18     19     1     0.538   0.0674        0.4206        0.687
##     22     15     1     0.502   0.0718        0.3792        0.664
##     25      9     2     0.390   0.0892        0.2494        0.611
##     28      5     1     0.312   0.0998        0.1669        0.584
##     29      4     1     0.234   0.1009        0.1007        0.545
##     41      2     1     0.117   0.0970        0.0231        0.593
```

Next, we will estimate the survival probabilities for stroke type:

```
KM_str_type2 <- survfit(Surv(time = time2,
                             event = status ==."dead" ) ~ stroke_type,
                        data = stroke)
summary(KM_str_type2)
```

```
## Call: survfit(formula = Surv(time = time2, event = status == "dead") ~
##     stroke_type, data = stroke)
##
##                  stroke_type=HS
## time n.risk n.event survival std.err lower 95% CI upper 95% CI
##    1     69      6    0.913   0.0339        0.8489        0.982
##    2     61      1    0.898   0.0365        0.8293        0.973
##    3     58      4    0.836   0.0453        0.7520        0.930
##    4     52      2    0.804   0.0489        0.7136        0.906
##    5     47      4    0.736   0.0554        0.6346        0.853
##    6     38      2    0.697   0.0589        0.5905        0.822
##    7     34      2    0.656   0.0621        0.5447        0.790
##    9     30      1    0.634   0.0638        0.5205        0.772
##   10     27      1    0.611   0.0656        0.4945        0.754
##   12     24      2    0.560   0.0693        0.4390        0.713
##   14     19      1    0.530   0.0717        0.4068        0.691
##   18     15      1    0.495   0.0751        0.3675        0.666
##   22     11      1    0.450   0.0806        0.3166        0.639
##   25      6      2    0.300   0.1019        0.1541        0.584
##   29      2      1    0.150   0.1176        0.0322        0.698
##
##                  stroke_type=IS
## time n.risk n.event survival std.err lower 95% CI upper 95% CI
##    1    144      3    0.979   0.0119        0.956        1.000
##    2    129      3    0.956   0.0174        0.923        0.991
##    4     78      2    0.932   0.0241        0.886        0.980
##    5     43      1    0.910   0.0318        0.850        0.975
##    6     27      1    0.876   0.0451        0.792        0.970
```

```
##    7   22    2   0.797   0.0676      0.675       0.941
##   12    9    2   0.620   0.1223      0.421       0.912
##   14    5    1   0.496   0.1479      0.276       0.890
##   28    3    1   0.331   0.1671      0.123       0.890
##   41    1    1   0.000     NaN         NA          NA
```

11.8 Plot the Survival Probability

The KM estimate provides the survival probabilities. We can plot these probabilities to look at the trend of survival over time. The plot provides

1. survival probability on the $y-axis$
2. time on the $x-axis$

```
ggsurvplot(KM_str_type2,
           data = stroke,
           risk.table = TRUE,
           linetype = c(1,4),
           tables.height = 0.3,
           pval = TRUE)
```

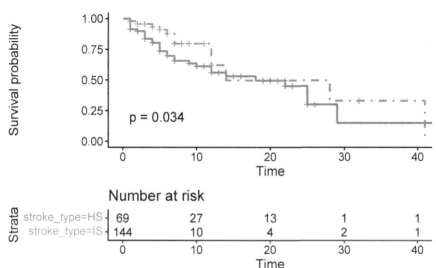

We can perform the Kaplan–Meier estimates for variable dm too:

```
KM_dm <- survfit(Surv(time = time2,
                      event = status == "dead" ) ~ dm,
                 data = stroke)
summary(KM_dm)
```

```
## Call: survfit(formula = Surv(time = time2, event = status == "dead") ~
##     dm, data = stroke)
##
##               dm=no
##  time n.risk n.event survival std.err lower 95% CI upper 95% CI
##     1    141       8    0.943  0.0195       0.9058        0.982
##     2    122       4    0.912  0.0242       0.8661        0.961
##     3    102       2    0.894  0.0268       0.8434        0.949
##     4     82       2    0.873  0.0303       0.8152        0.934
##     5     54       5    0.792  0.0441       0.7100        0.883
##     6     40       3    0.732  0.0524       0.6366        0.843
##     7     34       2    0.689  0.0575       0.5854        0.812
##    10     24       1    0.661  0.0619       0.5498        0.794
##    12     20       4    0.529  0.0771       0.3971        0.703
##    18     13       1    0.488  0.0812       0.3521        0.676
##    22      9       1    0.434  0.0884       0.2908        0.647
##    25      4       1    0.325  0.1149       0.1627        0.650
##    29      3       1    0.217  0.1171       0.0752        0.625
##
##               dm=yes
##  time n.risk n.event survival std.err lower 95% CI upper 95% CI
##     1     72       1    0.986  0.0138       0.9594        1.000
##     3     64       2    0.955  0.0253       0.9070        1.000
##     4     48       2    0.915  0.0367       0.8463        0.990
##     7     22       2    0.832  0.0653       0.7137        0.971
##     9     15       1    0.777  0.0811       0.6330        0.953
##    14      9       2    0.604  0.1248       0.4030        0.906
##    25      5       1    0.483  0.1471       0.2662        0.878
##    28      2       1    0.242  0.1860       0.0534        1.000
##    41      1       1    0.000     NaN           NA           NA
```

And then we can plot the survival estimates for patients with and without diabetes:

```
ggsurvplot(KM_dm,
           data = stroke,
           risk.table = TRUE,
           linetype = c(1,4),
```

```
tables.height = 0.3,
pval = TRUE)
```

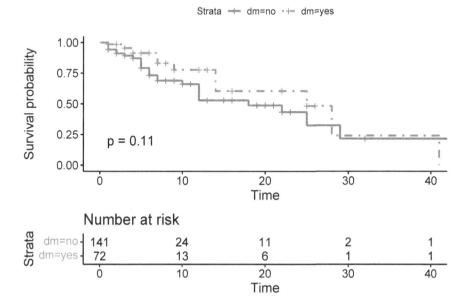

11.9 Comparing Kaplan–Meier Estimates across Groups

There are a number of available tests to compare the survival estimates between groups based on KM. The tests include:

1. log-rank (default)
2. peto-peto test

11.9.1 Log-rank test

From Kaplan–Meier survival curves, we could see the graphical representation of survival probabilities in different group over time. And to answer question if the survival estimates are different between levels or groups we can use statistical tests for example the log-rank and the peto-peto tests.

For all the test, the null hypothesis is that the survival estimates between levels or groups are not different. For example, to do that:

```
survdiff(Surv(time = time2,
              event = status == "dead") ~ stroke_type,
         data = stroke,
         rho = 0)
```

```
## Call:
## survdiff(formula = Surv(time = time2, event = status == "dead") ~
##      stroke_type, data = stroke, rho = 0)
##
##                     N Observed Expected (O-E)^2/E (O-E)^2/V
## stroke_type=HS   69      31     24.2      1.92      4.51
## stroke_type=IS  144      17     23.8      1.95      4.51
##
##   Chisq= 4.5  on 1 degrees of freedom, p= 0.03
```

The survival estimates between the stroke types (*IS* vs *HS* groups) are different at the level of 5% significance (p-value = 0.03).

And for the survival estimates based on diabetes status:

```
survdiff(Surv(time = time2,
              event = status == "dead") ~ dm,
         data = stroke,
         rho = 0)
```

```
## Call:
## survdiff(formula = Surv(time = time2, event = status == "dead") ~
##      dm, data = stroke, rho = 0)
##
##            N Observed Expected (O-E)^2/E (O-E)^2/V
## dm=no   141      35     29.8      0.919     2.54
## dm=yes   72      13     18.2      1.500     2.54
##
##   Chisq= 2.5  on 1 degrees of freedom, p= 0.1
```

The survival estimates between patients with and without diabetes (dm status *yes* vs *no* groups) are not different (p-value = 0.1).

11.9.2   Peto-peto test

We will be confident with our results if we obtain almost similar findings from other tests. So, now let's compare survival estimates using the peto-peto test.

This is the result for comparing survival estimates for stroke type using peto-peto test.

```
survdiff(Surv(time = time2,
              event = status == "dead") ~ stroke_type,
         data = stroke,
         rho = 1)
```

```
## Call:
## survdiff(formula = Surv(time = time2, event = status == "dead") ~
##      stroke_type, data = stroke, rho = 1)
##
##                    N Observed Expected (O-E)^2/E (O-E)^2/V
## stroke_type=HS   69    25.3     18.7      2.33      6.02
## stroke_type=IS  144    13.7     20.3      2.15      6.02
##
##   Chisq= 6  on 1 degrees of freedom, p= 0.01
```

This is the result for comparing survival estimates for diabetes status using peto-peto test.

```
survdiff(Surv(time = time2,
              event = status == "dead") ~ dm,
         data = stroke,
         rho = 1)
```

```
## Call:
## survdiff(formula = Surv(time = time2, event = status == "dead") ~
##      dm, data = stroke, rho = 1)
##
##            N Observed Expected (O-E)^2/E (O-E)^2/V
## dm=no    141    29.54    24.3      1.11      3.61
## dm=yes    72     9.41    14.6      1.85      3.61
##
##   Chisq= 3.6  on 1 degrees of freedom, p= 0.06
```

11.10 Semi-Parametric Models in Survival Analysis

One advantage of time-to-event data (from a cohort study) is the ability to estimate the hazard or risk to develop the event (outcome) of interest. However, the challenge in the cohort study is the presence of censoring. Censoring can happen due to

- patients leave the study (loss to follow-up) randomly
- patients do not experience the event even at the termination of the study

- patients are withdrawn from the study

In censored patients, we do not know exactly the time for them to develop the event.

To explore how to incorporate a regression model-like structure into the hazard function, we can model the hazard function using:

$$h(t) = \theta_0$$

The hazard function is a rate, and because of that it must be strictly positive. To constrain θ at greater than zero, we can parameterize the hazard function as:

$$h(t) = \exp^{\beta_0}$$

So for a covariate x the log-hazard function is:

$$ln[h(t.x)] = \beta_0 + \beta_1(x)$$

and the hazard function is

$$h(t.x) = exp^{\beta_0 + \beta_1(x)}$$

This is the exponential distribution which is one example of a fully parametric hazard function. Fully parametric models accomplish two goals simultaneously:

- It describes the basic underlying distribution of survival time (error component)
- It characterizes how that distribution changes as a function of the covariates (systematic component).

However, even though fully parametric models can be used to accomplish the above goals, the assumptions required for their error components may be unnecessarily stringent or unrealistic. One option is to have a fully parametric regression structure but leave their dependence on time unspecified. The models that utilize this approach are called semiparametric regression models.

11.10.1   Cox proportional hazards regression

If we take our dataset, for example, where want to compare the survival experience of stroke patients on different types of stroke (Ischemic stroke vs Hemorrhagic stroke), one form of a regression model for the hazard function that addresses the study goal is:

$$h(t, x, \beta) = h_0(t)r(x, \beta)$$

We can see that the hazard function is the product of two functions:

- The function, $h_0(t)$, characterizes how the hazard function changes as a function of survival time.

- The function, $r(x, \beta)$, characterizes how the hazard function changes as a function of subject covariates.

The $h_0(t)$ is frequently referred to as the baseline hazard function. Thus the baseline hazard function is, in some sense, a generalization of the intercept or constant term found in parametric regression models.

The hazard ratio (HR) depends only on the function $r(x, \beta)$. If the ratio function $HR(t, x_1, x_0)$ has a clear clinical interpretation then, the actual form of the baseline hazard function is of little importance.

With this parameterization the hazard function is

$$h(t, x, \beta) = h_o(t)exp^{x\beta}$$

and the hazard ratio is

$$HR(t, x_1, x_0) = exp^{\beta(x_1 - x_0)}$$

This model is referred to in the literature by a variety of terms, such as the Cox model, the Cox proportional hazards model or simply the proportional hazards model.

So, for example, if we have a covariate that is a dichotomous (binary), such as stroke type: coded as a value of $x_1 = 1$ and $x_0 = 0$, for HS and IS, respectively, then the hazard ratio becomes

$$HR(t, x_1, x_0) = exp^{\beta}$$

If the value of the coefficient is $\beta = ln(2)$, then the interpretation is that HS are dying at twice $(exp^{\beta} = 2)$ the rate of patients with IS.

11.10.2   Advantages of the Cox proportional hazards regression

If you remember that by using Kaplan–Meier (KM) analysis, we could estimate the survival probability. And using the log-rank or peto-peto test, we could compare the survival between categorical covariates. However, the disadvantages of KM include:

1. Need to categorize numerical variable to compare survival
2. It is a univariable analysis
3. It is a non-parametric analysis

We also acknowledge that the fully parametric regression models in survival analysis have stringent assumptions and distribution requirements. So, to overcome the limitations of the KM analysis and the fully parametric analysis, we can model our survival data using the semi-parametric **Cox proportional hazards regression**.

11.11   Estimation from Cox Proportional Hazards Regression

11.11.1   Simple Cox PH regression

Using our stroke dataset, we will estimate the parameters using the Cox PH regression. Remember, in our data, we have

1. the time variable : `time2`
2. the event variable : `status` and the event of interest is **dead**. Event classified other than dead are considered as censored.
3. date variables : date of admission (doa) and date of discharge (dod)
4. all other covariates

Now let's take stroke type as the covariate of interest:

```
stroke_stype <-
  coxph(Surv(time = time2,
             event = status == 'dead') ~ stroke_type,
                   data = stroke)
summary(stroke_stype)
```

```
## Call:
## coxph(formula = Surv(time = time2, event = status == "dead") ~
##     stroke_type, data = stroke)
##
##   n= 213, number of events= 48
##
##                 coef exp(coef) se(coef)      z Pr(>|z|)
## stroke_typeIS -0.6622    0.5157   0.3172 -2.088   0.0368 *
## ---
## Signif. codes:  0 '***' 0.001 '**' 0.01 '*' 0.05 '.' 0.1 ' ' 1
##
##               exp(coef) exp(-coef) lower .95 upper .95
## stroke_typeIS    0.5157      1.939     0.277    0.9602
##
## Concordance= 0.623  (se = 0.045 )
## Likelihood ratio test= 4.52  on 1 df,   p=0.03
## Wald test            = 4.36  on 1 df,   p=0.04
## Score (logrank) test = 4.48  on 1 df,   p=0.03
```

But for nicer output (in a data frame format), we can use `tidy()`. This will give us

- the estimate which is the log hazard. If you exponentiate it, you will get hazard ratio

- the standard error
- the p-value
- the confidence intervals for the log hazard

```
tidy(stroke_stype,
     conf.int = TRUE)
```

```
## # A tibble: 1 x 7
##    term          estimate std.error statistic p.value conf.low conf.high
##    <chr>            <dbl>     <dbl>     <dbl>   <dbl>    <dbl>     <dbl>
## 1 stroke_typeIS   -0.662     0.317    -2.09   0.0368   -1.28    -0.0406
```

The simple Cox PH model with covariate stroke type shows that the patients with IS has −0.0662 times the crude log hazard for death as compared to patients with HS (p-value = 0.0368).

The 95% confidence intervals for the crude log hazards are calculated by:

$$\hat{\beta} \pm 1.96 \times \widehat{SE}(\hat{\beta})$$

$$-0.662 \pm 1.96 \times 0.317 = -1.284, -0.041$$

```
tidy(stroke_stype,
     exponentiate = TRUE,
     conf.int = TRUE)
```

```
## # A tibble: 1 x 7
##    term          estimate std.error statistic p.value conf.low conf.high
##    <chr>            <dbl>     <dbl>     <dbl>   <dbl>    <dbl>     <dbl>
## 1 stroke_typeIS    0.516     0.317    -2.09   0.0368    0.277     0.960
```

Or we can get the crude hazard ratio (HR) by exponentiating the log HR. In this example, the simple Cox PH model with covariate stroke type shows that the patients with IS has 49% lower risk for stroke death as compared to patients with HS (p-value = 0.0368 and 95%CI0.277, 0.960).

The 95% confidence intervals for crude HR are calculated by

$$exp[\hat{\beta} \pm 1.96 \times \widehat{SE}(\hat{\beta})]$$

Hence, the lower bound for crude HR is $exp(-1.284) = 0.277$ and the upper bound for crude HR is $exp(-0.0041) = 0.996$ at 95% confidence.

Let's model the risk for stroke death for covariate gcs:

```
stroke_gcs <-
  coxph(Surv(time = time2,
             event = status == 'dead') ~ gcs,
             data = stroke)
summary(stroke_gcs)
```

```
## Call:
## coxph(formula = Surv(time = time2, event = status == "dead") ~
##     gcs, data = stroke)
##
##   n= 213, number of events= 48
##
##          coef exp(coef) se(coef)      z Pr(>|z|)
## gcs -0.17454   0.83984  0.03431 -5.087 3.63e-07 ***
## ---
## Signif. codes:  0 '***' 0.001 '**' 0.01 '*' 0.05 '.' 0.1 ' ' 1
##
##     exp(coef) exp(-coef) lower .95 upper .95
## gcs    0.8398      1.191    0.7852    0.8983
##
## Concordance= 0.763  (se = 0.039 )
## Likelihood ratio test= 26.01  on 1 df,   p=3e-07
## Wald test            = 25.88  on 1 df,   p=4e-07
## Score (logrank) test = 29.33  on 1 df,   p=6e-08
```

The simple Cox PH model with covariate gcs shows that with each one unit increase in gcs, the crude log hazard for death changes by a factor of -0.175.

```
tidy(stroke_gcs,
     exponentiate = TRUE,
     conf.int = TRUE)
```

```
## # A tibble: 1 x 7
##   term  estimate std.error statistic    p.value conf.low conf.high
##   <chr>    <dbl>     <dbl>     <dbl>      <dbl>    <dbl>     <dbl>
## 1 gcs      0.840    0.0343     -5.09 0.000000363    0.785     0.898
```

When we exponentiate the log HR, the simple Cox PH model shows that with each one unit increase in gcs, the crude risk for death decreases for about 16% and the of decrease are between $95\% CI (0.785, 0.898)$. The relationship between stroke death and gcs is highly significant (p-value < 0.0001) when not adjusting for other covariates.

By using `tbl_uvregression()` we can generate simple univariable model for all covariates in one line of code. In return, we get the crude HR for all the covariates of interest.

```
stroke %>%
  dplyr::select(time2, status, sex, dm, gcs, sbp, dbp, wbc,
                stroke_type, referral_from) %>%
  tbl_uvregression(
    method = coxph,
    y = Surv(time2, event = status == 'dead'),
    exponentiate = TRUE,
    pvalue_fun = ~style_pvalue(.x, digits = 3)
  ) %>%
  as_gt()
```

Characteristic	N	HR[1]	95% CI[1]	p-value
sex	213			
female		—	—	
male		0.71	0.37, 1.36	0.299
dm	213			
no		—	—	
yes		0.60	0.31, 1.13	0.112
gcs	213	0.84	0.79, 0.90	< 0.001
sbp	213	1.00	0.99, 1.01	0.617
dbp	213	1.00	0.98, 1.01	0.772
wbc	213	1.04	0.97, 1.11	0.270
stroke_type	213			
HS		—	—	
IS		0.52	0.28, 0.96	0.037
referral_from	213			
hospital		—	—	
non-hospital		0.58	0.32, 1.05	0.074

[1]HR = Hazard Ratio, CI = Confidence Interval

11.11.2 Multiple Cox PH regression

There are two primary reasons to include more than one covariate in the model. One of the primary reasons for using a regression model is to include multiple covariates to adjust statistically for possible imbalances in the observed data before making statistical inferences. In traditional statistical applications, it is called analysis of covariance, while in clinical and epidemiological investigations, it is often called control of confounding. The other reason is a statistically related issue where the inclusion of higher-order terms in a model representing interactions between covariates. These are also called effect modifiers.

Let's decide based on our clinical expertise and statistical significance, we would model a Cox PH model with these covariates.

- stroke_type
- gcs
- referral_from

The reason these covariates were selected was because we found that both gcs and stroke type are statistically significant. We also believe that the way patients are referred to hospital may indicate the severity of stroke. On the other hand, we assumed variables sex, sbp, dbp and wbc are not clinically important risk factors for stroke death.

In addition to that, we foresee that stroke type and death is mediated through gcs. For example, patients that suffer from hemorrhagic stroke will suffer more severe bleeding. This will lead to poorer gcs and poorer survival status. So, by adding both gcs and stroke, we can estimate the total effect from stroke type to death and the effect mediated through gcs.

To estimate to Cox PH model with stroke_type, gcs and referral_from:

```
stroke_mv <-
  coxph(Surv(time = time2,
             event = status == 'dead') ~ stroke_type +  gcs + referral_from,
        data = stroke)
tidy(stroke_mv, exponentiate = TRUE, conf.int = TRUE)
```

```
## # A tibble: 3 x 7
##    term              estimate std.error statistic p.value conf.low conf.high
##    <chr>                <dbl>     <dbl>     <dbl>   <dbl>    <dbl>     <dbl>
## 1 stroke_typeIS        0.835     0.345    -0.523 6.01e-1    0.424      1.64
## 2 gcs                  0.847    0.0358     -4.63 3.72e-6    0.790     0.909
## 3 referral_fromnon-hosp~ 0.824   0.322    -0.602 5.47e-1    0.439      1.55
```

or we may use `tbl_regression()` for a better output

```
tbl_regression(stroke_mv) %>%
  as_gt()
```

Characteristic	log(HR)[1]	95% CI[1]	p-value
stroke_type			
HS	—	—	
IS	−0.18	−0.86, 0.50	0.6
gcs	−0.17	−0.24, −0.10	< 0.001
referral_from			
hospital	—	—	
non-hospital	−0.19	−0.82, 0.44	0.5

[1]HR = Hazard Ratio, CI = Confidence Interval

and show the exponentiation of the log hazard ratio to obtain the hazard ratio

```
tbl_regression(stroke_mv, exponentiate = TRUE) %>%
  as_gt()
```

Characteristic	HR[1]	95% CI[1]	p-value
stroke_type			
HS	—	—	
IS	0.83	0.42, 1.64	0.6
gcs	0.85	0.79, 0.91	< 0.001
referral_from			
hospital	—	—	
non-hospital	0.82	0.44, 1.55	0.5

[1]HR = Hazard Ratio, CI = Confidence Interval

We would like to doubly confirm if the model with covariates stroke_type, gcs and referral_from and really statistically different from model with stroke type and referral from:

```
stroke_mv2 <-
  coxph(Surv(time = time2,
           event = status == 'dead') ~ stroke_type + referral_from,
       data = stroke)
tidy(stroke_mv, exponentiate = TRUE, conf.int = TRUE)
```

```
## # A tibble: 3 x 7
##   term          estimate std.error statistic p.value conf.low conf.high
##   <chr>            <dbl>     <dbl>     <dbl>   <dbl>    <dbl>     <dbl>
## 1 stroke_typeIS    0.835     0.345    -0.523 6.01e-1    0.424      1.64
```

```
## 2 gcs                      0.847    0.0358    -4.63 3.72e-6    0.790    0.909
## 3 referral_fromnon-hosp~   0.824    0.322     -0.602 5.47e-1    0.439    1.55
```

We can confirm this by running the likelihood ratio test between the two Cox PH models:

```
anova(stroke_mv, stroke_mv2, test = 'Chisq')
```

```
## Analysis of Deviance Table
## Cox model: response is  Surv(time = time2, event = status == "dead")
## Model 1: ~ stroke_type + gcs + referral_from
## Model 2: ~ stroke_type + referral_from
##    loglik Chisq Df Pr(>|Chi|)
## 1 -187.29
## 2 -198.08 21.57  1  3.412e-06 ***
## ---
## Signif. codes:  0 '***' 0.001 '**' 0.01 '*' 0.05 '.' 0.1 ' ' 1
```

And true enough, the two Cox PH modes are different (p-value < 0.0001). And we will choose the larger model.

11.12   Adding Interaction in the Model

Interaction in the model is an interesting phenomenon. To illustrate how we manage interaction term, let's start with a model with three covariates, gcs, stroke type and dm. In this model, based on clinical knowledge and curiosity, we would develop a two-way interaction term between gcs and stroke type. This interaction term (a product from gcs and stroke type) means the relationship between stroke type and risk for death is heterogenous in different values of gcs.

Let's assign stroke type as st and code it as either 1 (HS) and 0 (IS)

$$g(t, st, gsc, dm, \beta) = ln[h_0(t) + st\beta_1 + gcs\beta_2 + (st \times gcs)\beta_3 + dm\beta_4]$$

And the difference in the log hazard function becomes

$$[g(t, st = 1, gcs, dm, \beta) - g(t, st = 0, gcs, dm, \beta)]$$
$$= ln[h_0(t) + 1beta_1 + gcs\beta_2 + (1gcs)\beta_3 + dm\beta_4] -$$
$$ln[h_0(t) + 0beta_1 + gcs\beta_2 + (0gcs)\beta_3 + dm\beta_4]$$
$$= beta_1 + gcs\beta_3$$

This is a Cox PH main effect model. Main effect model means there is no interaction between variables in the model.

```
stroke_noia <-
  coxph(Surv(time = time2,
           event = status == 'dead') ~ stroke_type + gcs + dm,
        data = stroke)
tidy(stroke_noia, exponentiate = TRUE, conf.int = TRUE)
```

```
## # A tibble: 3 x 7
##    term          estimate std.error statistic   p.value conf.low conf.high
##    <chr>            <dbl>     <dbl>     <dbl>      <dbl>    <dbl>     <dbl>
## 1 stroke_typeIS    0.874    0.338    -0.400    0.689      0.450     1.69
## 2 gcs              0.843    0.0363   -4.68     0.00000282  0.785    0.906
## 3 dmyes            0.649    0.341    -1.27     0.204      0.333     1.27
```

To run model with an interaction for Cox PH model for example a two-way interaction between stroke type and gcs, we can run these codes:

```
stroke_ia <-
  coxph(Surv(time = time2,
           event = status == 'dead') ~ stroke_type + gcs + stroke_type:gcs + dm,
        data = stroke)
tbl_regression(stroke_ia, exponentiate = TRUE) %>%
  as_gt()
```

Characteristic	HR[1]	95% CI[1]	p-value
stroke_type			
HS	—	—	
IS	0.77	0.17, 3.41	0.7
gcs	0.84	0.76, 0.92	< 0.001
dm			
no	—	—	
yes	0.65	0.33, 1.28	0.2
stroke_type * gcs			
IS * gcs	1.01	0.88, 1.17	0.9

[1]HR = Hazard Ratio, CI = Confidence Interval

It appears that the p-value for the interaction term (a product of gcs and stroke type) is large (p-value = 0.9).

```
anova(stroke_ia, stroke_noia, test = 'Chisq')
```

```
## Analysis of Deviance Table
## Cox model: response is  Surv(time = time2, event = status == "dead")
## Model 1: ~ stroke_type + gcs + stroke_type:gcs + dm
## Model 2: ~ stroke_type + gcs + dm
##    loglik  Chisq Df Pr(>|Chi|)
## 1 -186.61
## 2 -186.63 0.0351  1     0.8514
```

And next, when we assess the likelihood ratio test to further confirm the importance of the interaction term. We observe the same result (p value = 0.851). And because of p-value of larger than 0.05 and we also believe that the interaction is not important in clinical setting, we have decided not to add the interaction term in the model. We always recommended to confirm the decision to add or remove independent variables including interaction term after discussion with subject matter experts, in this case, they could a stroke physician or a neurosurgeon.

11.13   The Proportional Hazard Assumption

11.13.1   Risk constant over time

The most important assumption in Cox PH regression is the proportionality of the hazards over time. It refers to the requirement that, the hazard functions are multiplicatively related and that their ratio is constant over survival time or it simply says that the estimated HR does not depend on time.

A check of the proportional hazards assumption can be done by looking at the parameter estimates $\beta_1, ..., \beta_q$ over time. And we can safely assume proportional hazards when the estimates don't vary much over time. In most settings, in order to test the PH assumption, we can employ two-step procedure for assessing:

• calculate covariate-specific tests and
• plot the scaled and smoothed-scaled Schoenfeld residuals obtained from the model.

11.13.2   Test for PH assumption

In many statistical software, the null hypothesis of constant regression coefficients can be tested, both globally as well as for each covariate. In R, this can be done using the cox.zph() function from the **survival** package.

```
stroke_zph <- cox.zph(stroke_mv, transform = 'km')
stroke_zph
```

```
##               chisq df    p
## stroke_type   1.38336 1 0.24
## gcs           0.00764 1 0.93
## referral_from 1.39355 1 0.24
## GLOBAL        1.63410 3 0.65
```

The global test is not significant (p value = 0.65), and the p-value for each of the co-variate is also larger than 0.05. These evidences support that the there risks are proportional over time.

```
stroke_zph_rank <- cox.zph(stroke_mv, transform = 'rank')
stroke_zph_rank
```

```
##               chisq df    p
## stroke_type   1.29 1 0.26
## gcs           1.62 1 0.20
## referral_from 1.86 1 0.17
## GLOBAL        3.05 3 0.38
```

11.13.3   Plots to assess PH assumption

We can plot these residuals

- deviance
- Schoenfeld
- scaled Schoenfeld

For example, let's start with plotting the residuals

```
ggcoxdiagnostics(stroke_mv, type = "deviance")
```

```
## Warning: `gather_()` was deprecated in tidyr 1.2.0.
## i Please use `gather()` instead.
## i The deprecated feature was likely used in the survminer package.
##   Please report the issue at <https://github.com/kassambara/survminer/issues>.
## This warning is displayed once every 8 hours.
## Call `lifecycle::last_lifecycle_warnings()` to see where this warning was
## generated.
```

```
## `geom_smooth()` using formula = 'y ~ x'
```

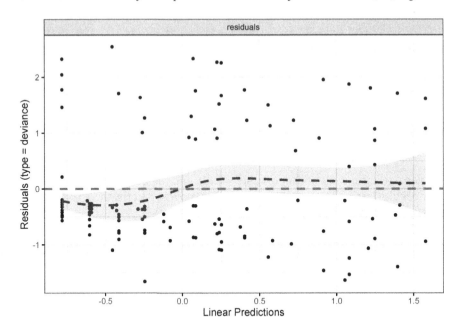

You may also plot the Schoenfeld residuals by replacing the type = deviance to type = Schoenfeld. You may refer to this link[1] for more details

```
plot(stroke_zph, var = "stroke_type")
```

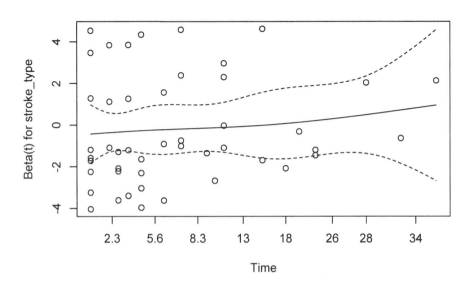

---

[1]http://pdf.medrang.co.kr/CSAM/2017/024/csam-24-583_suppl.pdf

• for gcs

```
plot(stroke_zph, var = "gcs")
```

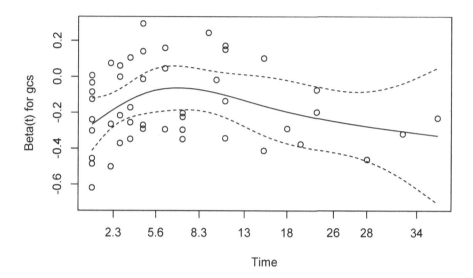

The plot for gcs shows possible violation of PH assumption. Even though, the coxzph() shows p value of larger than 0.05, there is a possibility that due to small sample size in the data, the PH test lost its power. However we believe that the violation is not severe.

• for referral type

```
plot(stroke_zph, var = "referral_from")
```

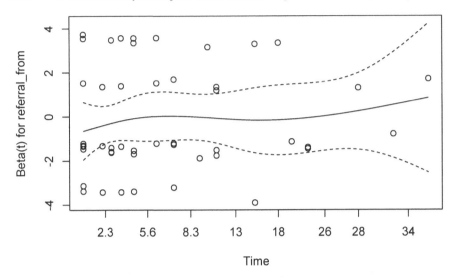

In the case of serious violation of proportionality of hazard, we can remedy using

1. stratified cox regression
2. extended cox regression using time-varying dependent variable
3. parametric survival analysis

11.14   Model Checking

11.14.1   Prediction from Cox PH model

From the Cox PH model, we can predict

1. the linear predictor
2. the risk
3. the expected number of events given the covariates and follow-up time

- The linear predictor

```
stroke_lp <- augment(stroke_mv, data = stroke)
stroke_lp %>%
  dplyr::select(gcs, stroke_type, referral_from, .fitted:.resid) %>%
  slice(1:10)


## # A tibble: 10 x 6
##      gcs stroke_type referral_from .fitted .se.fit  .resid
```

```
##     <dbl> <chr>    <chr>          <dbl>   <dbl>   <dbl>
## 1      15 IS       non-hospital  -0.785  0.365  -0.0192
## 2      15 IS       non-hospital  -0.785  0.365  -0.0192
## 3      11 HS       hospital       0.252  0.0545  0.970
## 4       3 IS       hospital       1.40   0.537   0.907
## 5      15 IS       non-hospital  -0.785  0.365  -0.0192
## 6       3 HS       hospital       1.58   0.341   0.888
## 7      11 IS       hospital       0.0716 0.361  -0.0453
## 8      15 IS       non-hospital  -0.785  0.365  -0.0192
## 9       6 HS       hospital       1.08   0.234   0.932
## 10     15 IS       non-hospital  -0.785  0.365  -0.0192
```

- The predicted risk which is the risk score $exp(lp)$ (*risk*),

```
risks <-
  augment(stroke_mv,
                data = stroke,
                type.predict = "risk")
risks %>%
  dplyr::select(status, gcs, stroke_type, referral_from, .fitted:.resid) %>%
  slice(1:10)
```

```
## # A tibble: 10 x 7
##     status   gcs stroke_type referral_from .fitted .se.fit  .resid
##     <chr>  <dbl> <chr>       <chr>           <dbl>   <dbl>   <dbl>
## 1  alive     15 IS          non-hospital    0.456  0.247  -0.0192
## 2  alive     15 IS          non-hospital    0.456  0.247  -0.0192
## 3  dead      11 HS          hospital        1.29   0.0618  0.970
## 4  dead       3 IS          hospital        4.05   1.08    0.907
## 5  alive     15 IS          non-hospital    0.456  0.247  -0.0192
## 6  dead       3 HS          hospital        4.85   0.751   0.888
## 7  alive     11 IS          hospital        1.07   0.374  -0.0453
## 8  alive     15 IS          non-hospital    0.456  0.247  -0.0192
## 9  dead       6 HS          hospital        2.95   0.401   0.932
## 10 alive     15 IS          non-hospital    0.456  0.247  -0.0192
```

- The expected is the expected number of events given the covariates and follow-up time ("expected"). The survival probability for a subject is equal to $exp(-expected)$.

```
expected <- augment(stroke_mv,
                data = stroke,
                type.predict = "expected")
```

```
expected %>%
  dplyr::select(status, gcs, stroke_type,
                referral_from, .fitted:.resid) %>%
  mutate(surv_prob = exp(-(.fitted))) %>%
  slice(1:10)
```

```
## # A tibble: 10 x 8
##    status   gcs stroke_type referral_from .fitted .se.fit  .resid surv_prob
##    <chr>  <dbl> <chr>       <chr>           <dbl>   <dbl>   <dbl>     <dbl>
## 1  alive    15 IS          non-hospital   0.0192 0.00801 -0.0192     0.981
## 2  alive    15 IS          non-hospital   0.0192 0.00801 -0.0192     0.981
## 3  dead     11 HS          hospital       0.0297 0.0209   0.970      0.971
## 4  dead      3 IS          hospital       0.0933 0.0853   0.907      0.911
## 5  alive    15 IS          non-hospital   0.0192 0.00801 -0.0192     0.981
## 6  dead      3 HS          hospital       0.112  0.0850   0.888      0.894
## 7  alive    11 IS          hospital       0.0453 0.0193  -0.0453     0.956
## 8  alive    15 IS          non-hospital   0.0192 0.00801 -0.0192     0.981
## 9  dead      6 HS          hospital       0.0680 0.0472   0.932      0.934
## 10 alive    15 IS          non-hospital   0.0192 0.00801 -0.0192     0.981
```

The Cox model is a relative risk model; predictions of type *linear predictor*, *risk*, and *terms* are all relative to the sample from which they came. By default, the reference value for each of these is the mean covariate within strata. Predictions of type *expected* incorporate the baseline hazard and are thus absolute instead of relative; the reference option has no effect on these.

11.14.2   Residuals from Cox PH model

Here, we will generate the

- martingale residuals
- deviance
- Schoenfeld
- dfbeta
- scaled schoenfeld

```
rmartingale <- residuals(stroke_mv, 'martingale')
rdeviance <- residuals(stroke_mv, 'deviance')
rschoenfeld <- residuals(stroke_mv, 'schoenfeld')
rdfbeta <- residuals(stroke_mv, 'dfbeta')
rscaled_sch <- residuals(stroke_mv, 'scaledsch')
```

11.14.3 Influential observations

We may check the $dfbetas$ residual. This is a residual that comes from a transformation of the score residual. It enables us to check the influence of dropping any single observation on parameter estimates. We may suspect influential observations when the $dfbetas$ residuals greater than 1.

```
ggcoxdiagnostics(stroke_mv,
                 type = "dfbetas",
                 point.size = 0,
                 hline.col = "black",
                 sline.col = "black") + geom_bar(stat = "identity")
```

```
## `geom_smooth()` using formula = 'y ~ x'
```

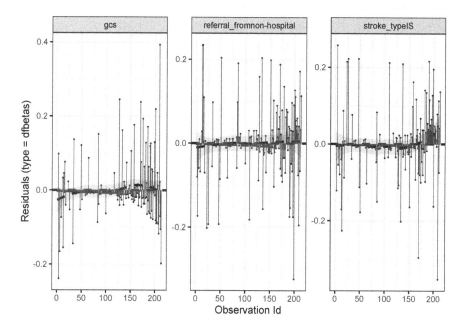

11.15 Plot the Adjusted Survival

The function `surv_adjustedcurves()` calculates while the function `ggadjustedcurves()` plots adjusted survival curves for the coxph model. The main idea behind this function is to present expected survival curves calculated based on Cox model separately for subpopulations.

```
# ggadjustedcurves(stroke_mv,
#                    data = stroke)
```

11.16 Presentation and Interpretation

The Cox PH model that we believe explains the risk for death among hospitalized acute stroke patients can be presented as below:

```
stroke_mv %>%
  tbl_regression(
    exponentiate = TRUE,
    pvalue_fun = ~style_pvalue(.x, digits = 3)
    ) %>%
  add_nevent(location = 'level') %>%
  bold_p(t = 0.10) %>%
  bold_labels() %>%
  as_gt()
```

Characteristic	Event N	HR[1]	95% CI[1]	p-value
stroke_type				
HS	31	—	—	
IS	17	0.83	0.42, 1.64	0.601
gcs	48	0.85	0.79, 0.91	< 0.001
referral_from				
hospital	29	—	—	
non-hospital	19	0.82	0.44, 1.55	0.547

[1]HR = Hazard Ratio, CI = Confidence Interval

11.17 Summary

In this chapter, we briefly describe the concept of survival analysis data, two common types of survival analysis (Kaplan–Meier and Cox PH regression) and provide skills to perform the analysis using R. We illustrate how to test for survival estimates for two samples and how to model the time-to-event data using single and multiple covariates in Cox PH regression. For further understanding of the survival analysis concepts and application, excellent texts include Survival Analysis: A Self-Learning Text (Kleinbaum and Klein, 2005) and Applied Survival Analysis: Regression Modeling of Time-to-Event Data (Lemeshow et al., 2008).

12

Parametric Survival Analysis

12.1 Objectives

At the end of the chapter, readers will be able

- to understand the basic concept of parametric survival analysis
- to understand the common parametric survival analysis models such as the exponential regression model and the Weibull survival mode.
- to perform the analysis for the exponential regression model and the Weibull regression model

12.2 Introduction

In survival analysis, the Cox proportional hazard (PH) regression is very popular to model the association between the time-to-event with covariates or independent variables. It is also a form of Generalized Linear Models. Cox PH regression is a semi-parametric survival analysis model.

The Cox Proportional Hazard model is the most popular technique to analysis the effects of covariates on survival time but under certain circumstances parametric models may offer advantages over Cox's model. In addition to Cox proportional hazard regression model, there is an additional class of survival models, called the parametric survival models. With parametric models such as linear regression, logistic regression and Poisson regression, the outcome is assumed to follow some distribution.

Researchers in medical sciences often tend to prefer semi-parametric instead of parametric models because of fewer assumptions but some comments recommended that under certain circumstances, parametric models estimate the parameter more efficient. In parametric models, we often use maximum likelihood procedures to estimate the unknown parameters and this technique and its interpretation are familiar for researchers. Also accelerated failure time can be used as relative risk with similar interpretation in Cox PH regression.

In the parametric survival models, the distribution of the outcome (i.e. the time to event) is specified in terms if unknown parameters. The interests in parametric models include:

- determining the acceleration factor and/or
- determining the hazard ratio.

The common parametric models include:

- Exponential survival model
- Weibull survival model and
- log-logistic survival model.

12.2.1   Advantages of parametric survival analysis models

A fully parametric model has some advantages (Lemeshow et al., 2008):

- full maximum likelihood may be used to estimate the parameters
- the estimated coefficients or transformations of them can provide clinically meaningful estimates of effect
- fitted values from the model can provide estimates of survival time
- residuals can be computed as differences between observed and predicted values of time

An analysis of censored time-to-event data using a fully parametric model can almost have the look and feel of a normal-errors linear regression analysis.

12.3   Parametric Survival Analysis Model

The shape of the survival or hazard curve is informative of the process and provides a link to substantive issues. Parametric models mean the outcome is assumed to follow some distributions. This also means that the outcome follows some family of distributions of similar form **BUT** with unknown parameters. In parametric survival analysis all parts of the model are specified, both the hazard function and the effect of any covariates.

The strength of this is that estimation is easier and estimated survival curves are smoother as they draw information from the whole data. The main drawback to parametric methods is that they require extra assumptions that may not be appropriate. Parametric models have proportional hazard metrics and accelerated failure time (AFT) metrics. AFT models allow covariates to predict survival. Often, no analytic solution for the MLE exists. In such cases, a numerical approach must be taken. A popular method is to use Newton Raphson.

Again, a parametric survival model is one of which survival time (the outcome) is assumed to follow a known distribution. The parametric models specify the baseline hazard and the baseline hazard indicates which model to be used, for example:

1. **Weibull model**
2. Log-logistic model
3. Log-normal model
4. **Exponential model**
5. Generalized Gamma model

For parametric survival models, time is assumed to follow some distribution whose probability density function $f(t)$ can be expressed in terms of unknown parameters. Once a probability density function is specified for survival time, the corresponding survival and hazard functions can be determined.

The survival function can also be expressed in terms of hazard function by exponentiating the negative cumulative hazard function. Probability density function can also be expressed as the product of the hazard and the survival function, $f(t) = h(t)S(t)$

Many parametric models are **Accelerated Failure Time (AFT)** models rather than **Proportional Hazard** models. And remember, *Constant Hazard* fulfills *Proportional Hazard* assumption, but *Proportional Hazard* does not mean a model has *Constant Hazard*.

12.3.1 Proportional hazard parametric models

Parametric models can be presented either as a **proportional hazard models** or **accelerated failure time (AFT)** models. Parametric models that have both the proportional hazards models and accelerated failure time models are:

1. Exponential model
2. Weibull model

If we take the Exponential model as an example, in the exponential survival model with a single covariate, X then the hazard function for the proportional hazard model is:

$$h(t) = \exp^{(\beta_0 + \beta_1 x)}$$
$$h(t) = \exp^{\beta_0} \exp^{\beta_1 x}$$
$$h(t) = h_0 \exp^{\beta_1 x}$$

12.3.2 Accelerated failure time model (AFT) models

Again, if we take the Exponential model with a single covariate, X then the hazard function for the AFT model is

$$h(t) = \frac{1}{(\exp^{\alpha_0 + \alpha_1 x})}$$
$$h(t) = \exp^{\alpha_0} \exp^{\alpha_1 x}$$
$$h(t) = h_0 \exp^{-\alpha_1 x}$$

A convenient and plausible way to characterize the distribution of time to event, denoted T, as a function of a single covariate is via the equation:

$$T = \exp^{\beta_0 + \beta_1 x} \times \epsilon$$

For the exponential model, these are equivalent, but this is not true in general. In other parametric models, it is possible for a model to be proportional hazard models but not AFT, or AFT but not proportional hazard models, or both, or neither.

Because time must be positive, then:

1. the systematic component, $\exp^{\beta_0 + \beta_1 x}$ must be positive
2. the error component ϵ must also be positive

We can linearize the model, by taking the natural log of each side of the equation. And, now it becomes:

$$ln(T) = \beta_0 + \beta_1 x + \epsilon^*$$

The error component, ϵ^* can follow different distributions. If the error component follows the exponential distribution, then we call the model as the exponential regression model. Other possible distribution includes Weibull regression model, lognormal model, log-logistics and others.

Survival time models that can be linearized by taking logs are called accelerated failure time models. The effect of covariate is multiplicative (proportional) with respect to survival time. Whereas, for the PH models, the assumption is that; the effect of covariates is multiplicative with respect to hazard.

12.4   Analysis

This study was conducted from the latest release data from the 2017 submission of the SEER database (1973 to 2015 data) of the National Cancer Institute. Patients with a diagnosis of AO were selected from the SEER database using the International Classification of Diseases for Oncology, Third Edition (ICD-O-3) histology code 9451. There are 1824 patients diagnosed with AO in this dataset.

12.4.1   Dataset

The dataset contains all variables of our interest. For the purpose of this assignment, we want to explore prognostic factor association of age, surgery status and marital status with the survival of AO patients. The variables in the dataset as follow:

- age : biological age at the beginning of the study. This data in numerical values.
- surgery : is the patient has undergone surgery. Coded as "Yes" and "No"
- marital : Marital status at diagnosis. Coded as "single", "married", or "separated/divorced/widowed".
- survivaltime : survival time in month. This data is in numerical values.
- status : survival status coded as "1 = died" and "0 = censored"

12.4.2   Set the environment

We use these packages:

- **here** to specify the location of the working directory
- **tidyverse** for exploratory data analysis, data wrangling and plotting.
- **gtsummary** to provide nice statistical tables
- **broom** to provide clean and polish table from the estimates
- **flexsurve** to perform flexible parametric survival analysis models for time-to-event data, including the generalized gamma, the generalized F and the Royston-Parmar spline model, and extensible to user-defined distributions.
- **SurvRefCensCov** to transforms output-based Weibull distribution to a more natural parameterization.

```
library(here)
```

```
## here() starts at C:/Users/drkim/Downloads/multivar_data_analysis/multivar_data_analysis
```

```
library(tidyverse)
```

```
## -- Attaching core tidyverse packages ----------------------- tidyverse 2.0.0 --
## v dplyr      1.1.1     v readr     2.1.4
## v forcats    1.0.0     v stringr   1.5.0
## v ggplot2    3.4.2     v tibble    3.2.1
## v lubridate  1.9.2     v tidyr     1.3.0
## v purrr      1.0.1
## --          Conflicts          ------------------------------------------
tidyverse_conflicts() --
## x dplyr::filter() masks stats::filter()
## x dplyr::lag()    masks stats::lag()
```

```
##     i     Use      the     conflicted     package     (<http://conflicted.r-
lib.org/>) to force all conflicts to become errors
```

```
library(gtsummary)
library(broom)
library(flexsurv)
```

```
## Loading required package: survival
```

```
library(SurvRegCensCov)
```

```
## Registered S3 method overwritten by 'SurvRegCensCov':
##    method    from
##    print.src dplyr
```

12.4.3   Read dataset

```
d1 <- read_csv(here('data','survivaloa.csv'))
```

```
## Rows: 1824 Columns: 8
## -- Column specification -------------------------------------------------
---
## Delimiter: ","
## chr (5): marital, sex, surgery, race, first
## dbl (3): age, status, survivaltime
##
## i Use `spec()` to retrieve the full column specification for this data.
## i Specify the column types or set `show_col_types = FALSE` to quiet this message.
```

12.4.4   Data wrangling

We will select only these variables to simplify our model-building process:

- age
- surgery
- marital
- survivaltime
- status

And then we will convert all character variables to factor variables.

```
d1<- d1 %>%
  dplyr::select(age, surgery, marital, survivaltime, status) %>%
  mutate_if(is.character, as.factor)
glimpse(d1)
```

```
## Rows: 1,824
## Columns: 5
## $ age          <dbl> 4, 4, 4, 5, 5, 5, 6, 6, 6, 8, 9, 11, 11, 11, 11, 12, 13, ~
## $ surgery      <fct> Yes, Yes, Yes, Yes, No, No, Yes, Yes, Yes, Yes, Yes, Yes,~
## $ marital      <fct> Single, Single, Single, Single, Single, Single, Single, S~
## $ survivaltime <dbl> 290, 9, 10, 141, 12, 54, 161, 60, 11, 8, 15, 298, 83, 15,~
## $ status       <dbl> 0, 1, 1, 0, 1, 1, 0, 0, 1, 1, 1, 0, 0, 1, 1, 0, 1, 0, 1, ~
```

12.4.5 Exploratory data analysis (EDA)

We will do simple eda

```
d1 %>%
  mutate(status = recode(status,"0" = "Censored", "1" = "Death")) %>%
  tbl_summary(by = status,
              statistic = list(all_continuous() ~ "{mean} ({sd})",
                               all_categorical() ~ "{n} ({p}%)"),
              type = list(where(is.logical) ~ "categorical"),
              label = list(age ~ "Age (in years old)",
                           surgery ~ "Surgery Status",
                           marital~"Marital Status", survivaltime ~ "Time
↪ (month)"),
              missing_text = "Missing") %>%
  modify_caption("**Table 1. Patient Characteristic**")  %>%
  modify_header(label ~ "**Variable**") %>%
  modify_spanning_header(c("stat_1", "stat_2") ~ "**Survival Status**") %>%
  modify_footnote(all_stat_cols() ~ "Mean (SD) or Frequency (%)") %>%
  bold_labels() %>%
  as_gt()
```

	Survival Status	
Variable	**Censored**, N = 835[1]	**Death**, N = 989[1]
Age (in years old)	45 (13)	52 (16)
Surgery Status	774 (93%)	835 (84%)
Marital Status		
Married	531 (64%)	606 (61%)
Separated/divorced/widowed	96 (11%)	174 (18%)
Single	208 (25%)	209 (21%)
Time (month)	83 (65)	38 (42)

[1]Mean (SD) or Frequency (%)

12.4.6   Exponential survival model

We can use the `survreg()` from **survival** package. However `survreg()` only perform estimation for AFT metric.

```
exp.mod.aft <- survreg(Surv(survivaltime, status) ~ age + marital + surgery,
                       data = d1, dist = 'exponential')
summary(exp.mod.aft)
```

```
##
## Call:
## survreg(formula = Surv(survivaltime, status) ~ age + marital +
##     surgery, data = d1, dist = "exponential")
##                                    Value Std. Error      z       p
## (Intercept)                       6.6348     0.1601  41.45 < 2e-16
## age                              -0.0487     0.0025 -19.50 < 2e-16
## maritalSeparated/divorced/widowed -0.0609    0.0871  -0.70 0.48458
## maritalSingle                    -0.3068     0.0823  -3.73 0.00019
## surgeryYes                        0.5250     0.0879   5.97 2.4e-09
##
## Scale fixed at 1
##
## Exponential distribution
## Loglik(model)= -5401.2   Loglik(intercept only)= -5614.4
##   Chisq= 426.47 on 4 degrees of freedom, p= 5.3e-91
## Number of Newton-Raphson Iterations: 5
## n= 1824
```

12.4.7 Weibull (accelerated failure time)

We first start with estimating a Weibull parametric survival model which will return an accelerated failure metric:

To do this, we will be using the survreg() function

```
wei.mod.aft <- survreg(Surv(survivaltime, status) ~ age + surgery + marital,
                    data = d1, dist = 'weibull')
summary(wei.mod.aft)
```

```
##
## Call:
## survreg(formula = Surv(survivaltime, status) ~ age + surgery +
##     marital, data = d1, dist = "weibull")
##                                       Value Std. Error      z        p
## (Intercept)                          6.82050    0.19724  34.58  < 2e-16
## age                                 -0.05270    0.00305 -17.26  < 2e-16
## surgeryYes                           0.62515    0.10897   5.74  9.7e-09
## maritalSeparated/divorced/widowed   -0.10037    0.10713  -0.94   0.3488
## maritalSingle                       -0.35437    0.10184  -3.48   0.0005
## Log(scale)                           0.20727    0.02577   8.04  8.8e-16
##
## Scale= 1.23
##
## Weibull distribution
## Loglik(model)= -5365.4   Loglik(intercept only)= -5533.9
##  Chisq= 336.93 on 4 degrees of freedom, p= 1.2e-71
## Number of Newton-Raphson Iterations: 5
## n= 1824
```

However, the parameters estimated from survreg() does not make clinical sense. So, we will convert to log hazard ratio, hazard ratio and estimated time ratio. To do this, we will use the ConvertWeibull() to convert the Weibull PH to Weibul AFT model

```
ConvertWeibull(wei.mod.aft, conf.level = 0.95)
```

```
## $vars
##                                       Estimate           SE
## lambda                             0.003912012  0.0007814675
## gamma                              0.812800295  0.0209455354
## age                                0.042835914  0.0025361397
## surgeryYes                        -0.508122220  0.0879913395
## maritalSeparated/divorced/widowed  0.081578034  0.0869994355
## maritalSingle                      0.288029086  0.0826554798
##
```

```
## $HR
##                                              HR        LB        UB
## age                                   1.0437666 1.0385912 1.0489678
## surgeryYes                            0.6016242 0.5063222 0.7148644
## maritalSeparated/divorced/widowed     1.0849979 0.9149025 1.2867167
## maritalSingle                         1.3337961 1.1343132 1.5683606
##
## $ETR
##                                             ETR        LB        UB
## age                                   0.9486630 0.9430040 0.9543559
## surgeryYes                            1.8685265 1.5091765 2.3134412
## maritalSeparated/divorced/widowed     0.9045057 0.7331977 1.1158390
## maritalSingle                         0.7016179 0.5746698 0.8566096
```

Or we can simply use flexsurv() to obtain the log time ratio and time ratio.

```
wei.mod.aft <- flexsurvreg(Surv(survivaltime, status) ~ age + surgery + marital,
                           data = d1, dist = 'weibull')
wei.mod.aft
```

```
## Call:
## flexsurvreg(formula = Surv(survivaltime, status) ~ age + surgery +
##     marital, data = d1, dist = "weibull")
##
## Estimates:
##                                    data mean   est        L95%       U95%
## shape                                    NA    8.13e-01   7.73e-01   8.55e-01
## scale                                    NA    9.16e+02   6.23e+02   1.35e+03
## age                                4.89e+01   -5.27e-02  -5.87e-02  -4.67e-02
## surgeryYes                         8.82e-01    6.25e-01   4.12e-01   8.39e-01
## maritalSeparated/divorced/widowed  1.48e-01   -1.00e-01  -3.10e-01   1.10e-01
## maritalSingle                      2.29e-01   -3.54e-01  -5.54e-01  -1.55e-01
##                                    se         exp(est)   L95%       U95%
## shape                              2.10e-02         NA         NA         NA
## scale                              1.81e+02         NA         NA         NA
## age                                3.05e-03   9.49e-01   9.43e-01   9.54e-01
## surgeryYes                         1.09e-01   1.87e+00   1.51e+00   2.31e+00
## maritalSeparated/divorced/widowed  1.07e-01   9.05e-01   7.33e-01   1.12e+00
## maritalSingle                      1.02e-01   7.02e-01   5.75e-01   8.57e-01
##
## N = 1824,  Events: 989,  Censored: 835
## Total time at risk: 106252
## Log-likelihood = -5365.418, df = 6
## AIC = 10742.84
```

12.4.7.1 Interpretation for accelerated failure time

The interpretation of the parameters is as below:

- The estimated log time ratio to die for every increment of 1 year of age was -0.0527. The Acceleration Factor (AF) or Time Ratio (TR) is $\exp(-0.0527)$ which equals 0.949. It means that for every 1 year increase in age, OA patients will die earlier (a factor of 0.949). Or, we can say for every 1 year increase in age, the survival time for OA patients will be significantly shorter by 5.1% when adjusted for surgery status and marital status. The reduction in survival in OA patients could range between 4.6% and 5.7% (Adj. TR = 0.949, 95% CI = 0.943, 0.954).

- The estimated log time ratio to die in OA patients who underwent surgery (in comparison to those who did not) was 0.625. The Acceleration Factor (AF) or Time Ratio (TR) is $\exp(0.625)$ which equals 1.87. The survival time for OA patients who underwent surgery was estimated to be 1.87% times longer than that of patients who did not undergo surgery. Or, it also means, the survival time among OA patients who underwent surgery was 87.0% longer than those who did not go for surgery, when adjusted for age and marital status. The increase duration of survival ranges between 51.0% and 131.0% (Adj. TR = 1.87, 95% CI = 1.51, 2.31)

- The estimated log time ratio to die in subjects who were single (in comparison to those who were married) was -0.354. The Acceleration Factor (AF) or Time Ratio (TR) is $\exp(-0.354)$ which equals 0.702. The survival time for OA patients who were single is shorter, estimated to be about a factor of 70.2% than OA patients who were married. The survival time among OA patients who were single was shorter by 29.8% when adjusted for surgery status and age. The survival shortened between 14.3% and 42.5% (Adj. TR = 0.702, 95% CI = 0.575, 0.857).

- The estimated log time ratio to die in subjects who were separated or divorced or widowed (in comparison to those who are married) was -0.100. The Acceleration Factor (AF) or Time Ratio (TR) is $\exp(-0.100)$ which equals 0.905. This shows that the survival of OA patients who were separated or divorced or widowed was 90.5% as compared to OA patients who were married. The survival time in OA patients who were separated or divorced or widowed was shorter by 9.5% when adjusted for surgery status and age. The reduction is survival time ranged between 26.7% and 12.0% (Adj. TR = 0.905, 95% CI = 0.733, 1.12).

12.4.8 Weibull (proportional hazard)

In contrast to AFT metric, the `flexsurvreg()` could convert the estimation to proportional hazard (PH) metric. Below, we will obtain the estimate for log hazard ratio and the hazard ratio with their 95% confidence intervals.

```
wei.mod.ph <- flexsurvreg(Surv(survivaltime, status) ~ age + surgery + marital,
                          data = d1, dist = 'weibullPH')
wei.mod.ph
```

```
## Call:
## flexsurvreg(formula = Surv(survivaltime, status) ~ age + surgery +
##     marital, data = d1, dist = "weibullPH")
##
## Estimates:
##                                     data mean   est        L95%        U95%
## shape                               NA         0.812800   0.772768    0.854907
## scale                               NA         0.003912   0.002645    0.005786
## age                                 48.937500  0.042836   0.037872    0.047799
## surgeryYes                          0.882127  -0.508122  -0.680582   -0.335662
## maritalSeparated/divorced/widowed   0.148026   0.081578  -0.088939    0.252095
## maritalSingle                       0.228618   0.288029   0.126030    0.450028
##                                     se         exp(est)   L95%        U95%
## shape                               0.020945   NA         NA          NA
## scale                               0.000781   NA         NA          NA
## age                                 0.002532   1.043767   1.038599    1.048960
## surgeryYes                          0.087991   0.601624   0.506322    0.714865
## maritalSeparated/divorced/widowed   0.087000   1.084998   0.914901    1.286718
## maritalSingle                       0.082654   1.333796   1.134316    1.568356
##
## N = 1824,  Events: 989,  Censored: 835
## Total time at risk: 106252
## Log-likelihood = -5365.418, df = 6
## AIC = 10742.84
```

12.4.8.1 Interpretation for proportional hazard metric

- The log g hazard ratio for death among OA patients who underwent surgery to those who did not go for surgery was -0.508 which equals to hazard ratio of 0.60. It means the hazard for death was 39.9% lower in OA patients who went for surgery as compared to OA patients who did not undergo surgery, adjusted for age and marital status. The reduction in risk for death ranges between 29% and 50% (Adj. HR = 0.601, 95% CI = 0.50,0.71).

- An increase of 1 year of age would increase the log hazard by 0.043 or the risk (hazard) for death by 4.4% when adjusted for marital status and surgery status. The risk for death could increase between 3.9% and 4.9% (Adj. HR = 1.043, 95% CI = 1.039, 1.049).

- OA Patients who were separated or widowed or divorced had higher risk (hazard) for death by 8.5% as compared to OA patients who were married, when adjusted for age and surgery status. The risk for death could be lower by 9% or higher by 29% (Adj. HR = 1.085, 95% CI = 0.91, 1.29).

- OA patients who were single had an increase risk for death (by 33%) as compared to OA patients who were married, when adjusted for age and surgery status. The increase in the risk for death for single OA patients range between 13% and 57% (Adj. HR = 1.33, 95% CI = 1.13, 1.568).

12.4.9   Model adequacy for Weibull distribution

```
WeibullDiag(Surv(time = d1$survivaltime, event = d1$status == 1) ~ surgery,
            data = d1)
```

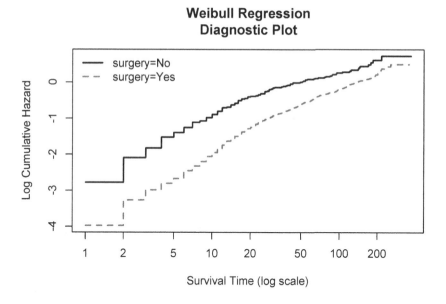

Weibull Regression Diagnostic Plot

From the Weibull regression diagnostic plot, we can see that the lines for surgery status (yes and no) are generally parallel and linear in its scale. Thus, we can assume that the Weibull model is fit.

```
WeibullDiag(Surv(time = d1$survivaltime, event = d1$status == 1) ~ marital,
            data = d1)
```

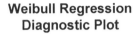

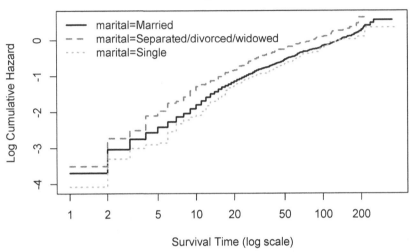

The Weibull regression diagnostic plot for marital status also shows rather parallel and linear lines. Again, we can assume that the Weibull model is fit.

12.5 Summary

In this chapter, we learned briefly the concept of parametric survival analysis. We are also shown how to perform parametric survival analysis for the exponential regression model and the Weibull regression model. In each model, we further illustrate the accelerated failure time (AFT) and proportional hazed (PH) metrics. For more understanding, we recommend Survival Analysis: A Self-Learning Text book (Kleinbaum and Klein, 2005) and Applied Survival Analysis: Regression Modeling of Time-to-Event Data book (Lemeshow et al., 2008).

13

Introduction to Missing Data Analysis

13.1 Objectives

At the end of the chapter, readers will be able to:

- To perform a simple imputation
- To perform a single imputation
- To perform a multiple imputation

13.2 Introduction

Missing data can significantly affect the performance of predictive risk modeling, an important technique for developing medical guidelines. The two most commonly used strategies for managing missing data are to impute or delete values, and the former can cause bias, while the later can cause both bias and loss of statistical power. Several techniques designed to deal with missing data are described and applied to an illustrative example. These methods include complete-case analysis, available-case analysis, as well as single and multiple imputation.

Researchers should report the details of missing data and appropriate methods for dealing with missing values should be incorporated into the data analysis.

13.3 Types of Missing Data

Missing data is quite a common issue in research. The causes of missing data should always be investigated and more data should be collected if possible. There are three types of missing data:

1. Missing completely at random (MCAR)

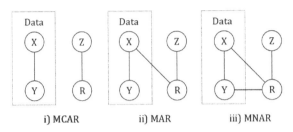

Source: Modified from Schafer and Graham (2002).

FIGURE 13.1
Illustration of missing data mechanism for the three types of missing data. The data is made up of X and Y. X represents a variable with completely observed values, Y represents a variable with missing values, Z represents a cause of missing values and R represents an indicator variable that identify missing and observed values in Y, in other words, the missingness.

2. Missing at random (MAR)
3. Missing not at random (MNAR)

Missing data is classified as MCAR if the missingness is unrelated to the data. For example, medical records that are lost due to flood and laboratory equipment malfunction, Z. In other words, the data is missing totally by chance. We can relate this example to Figure 13.1, the missingness, R is not related to the data itself, which is a combination of variables with completely observed values, X and variables with partly missing values, Y. MCAR is ideal and more convenient, though MAR is more common and realistic.

Missing data is said to be MAR if the missingness is related to other values that we completely observed, but not to the variable with missing values itself. For example, an older person is more likely to complete a survey compared to the younger person. So, the missingness is related to age, a variable that has been observed in the data. Similarly, if information on income is more likely to be missing for older individuals as they are more cautious to reveal a sensitive information as opposed to younger individuals. Thus, the missingness is related to age, which should be a variable that we have collected during the survey. The similarity between the two examples is that we completely observed the variable age. Another example of MAR is missing a certain variable due to the old medical form do not include this information in the form. However, a new updated medical form include this information. As the missingness is not related to the variable with missing values itself and we have the information whether the patients use an old or a new medical form, we can classify this missingness as MAR. We can see from all the examples that the missingness, R is related to other variables that we completely observed, X, but not to the variable with missing values itself, Y as illustrated in Figure 13.1.

Lastly, the missing data is considered MNAR if the missingness is related to the variable with missing values itself and other variables with completely observed values as well. Also, the missingness is considered MNAR if the causes completely unknown to us. In other words, we can not logically deduce that the missing data fit MCAR or MAR types. For example, missing a weight information for an obese individuals as the normal weighing scale may not able to weigh the individuals. Thus, according to 13.1, the pattern of missingness is considered MNAR as the missingness, R is related the variable with partly missing values itself, Y. However, we can never be sure of this without a further investigation about the mechanism of missingness and its causes. MNAR is the most problematic type among the three. There are a few approaches to differentiate between MCAR and MAR-MNAR. However, an approach to differentiate between MAR and MNAR has yet to be proposed. Thus, we need to use a logical reasoning to differentiate between the two types.

Alternatively, Figure 13.1 can be represented mathematically as follows:

$$MCAR : P(R|Z)$$
$$MAR : P(R|X, Z)$$
$$MNAR : P(R|X, Y, Z)$$

In MCAR, the missingness is completely related to the cause of missing data, Z, which is unrelated to variables with completely observed values, X and variables with missing values, Y. However, MAR allows the missingness to be related to X, on top of Z. Additionally, MNAR requires the missingness related to X, Y, and Z.

13.4 Preliminaries

13.4.1 Packages

We will use these packages:

- **mice**: for the single and multiple imputation
- **VIM**: for missing data exploration
- **naniar**: for missing data exploration
- **tidyverse**: for data wrangling and manipulation
- **gtsummary**: to provide a nice result in a table

```
library(mice)
library(VIM)
library(naniar)
library(tidyverse)
library(gtsummary)
```

13.4.2   Dataset

We going to use the coronary dataset that we used previously in linear regression chapter. However, this dataset have been altered to generate a missing values in it.

```
coroNA <- read_csv(here::here('data', "coronaryNA.csv"))
```

Next, we going to transform the all the character variables into a factor. `mutate_if()` will recognize all character variables and transform it into a factor.

```
coroNA <-
  coroNA %>%
  mutate_if(is.character, as.factor)
summary(coroNA)
```

```
##       age            race           chol           id            cad
##  Min.   :33.00   chinese:31   Min.   :4.000   Min.   :   1.0   cad   : 37
##  1st Qu.:43.00   indian :45   1st Qu.:5.362   1st Qu.: 901.5   no cad:163
##  Median :48.00   malay  :49   Median :6.050   Median :2243.5
##  Mean   :48.02   NA's   :75   Mean   :6.114   Mean   :2218.3
##  3rd Qu.:53.00                3rd Qu.:6.875   3rd Qu.:3346.8
##  Max.   :62.00                Max.   :9.350   Max.   :4696.0
##  NA's   :85                   NA's   :33
##       sbp             dbp             bmi          gender
##  Min.   : 88.0   Min.   : 56.00   Min.   :28.99   man   :100
##  1st Qu.:115.0   1st Qu.: 72.00   1st Qu.:36.10   woman:100
##  Median :126.0   Median : 80.00   Median :37.80
##  Mean   :130.2   Mean   : 82.31   Mean   :37.45
##  3rd Qu.:144.0   3rd Qu.: 92.00   3rd Qu.:39.20
##  Max.   :187.0   Max.   :120.00   Max.   :45.03
##
```

Missing data in R is denoted by NA. Further information about NA can be assessed by typing ?NA in the RStudio console. As seen above, the three variables; age, race and chol have missing values. We can further confirm this using a anyNA().

```
anyNA(coroNA)
```

```
## [1] TRUE
```

True indicates the presence of missing values in our data. Thus, we can further explore the missing values in our data.

13.5   Exploring Missing Data

The total percentage of missing values in our data is 10.7%.

```
prop_miss(coroNA)
```

```
## [1] 0.1072222
```

Percentage of missing data by variable:

```
miss_var_summary(coroNA)
```

```
## # A tibble: 9 x 3
##    variable n_miss pct_miss
##    <chr>     <int>    <dbl>
## 1 age          85     42.5
## 2 race         75     37.5
## 3 chol         33     16.5
## 4 id            0        0
## 5 cad           0        0
## 6 sbp           0        0
## 7 dbp           0        0
## 8 bmi           0        0
## 9 gender        0        0
```

Both `prop_miss()` and `miss_var_summary()` are from `naniar` package. Subsequently, We can explore the pattern of missing data using `aggr()` function from VIM. The `numbers` and `prop` arguments indicate that we want the missing information on the y-axis of the plot to be in number not proportion.

```
aggr(coroNA, numbers = TRUE, prop = FALSE)
```

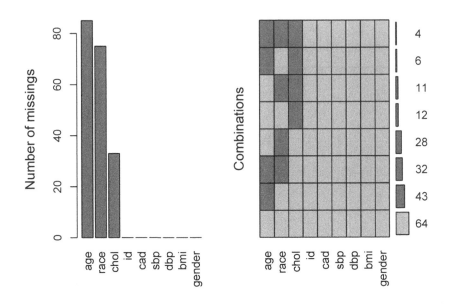

The labels on x-axis are according to the column names in the dataset. In term of pattern of missingness, about 43 observation are missing age values alone.

Similarly, the pattern of missing data can be explored through md.pattern() from mice package. The plot argument is set to FALSE since the plot is reflective of the pattern of missing data matrix below. To see the plot, the plot argument should be set to TRUE.

```
md.pattern(coroNA, plot = FALSE)
```

```
##     id cad sbp dbp bmi gender chol race age
## 64   1   1   1   1   1      1    1    1   0
## 43   1   1   1   1   1      1    1    0   1
## 28   1   1   1   1   1      1    1    0   1   1
## 32   1   1   1   1   1      1    1    0   0   2
## 12   1   1   1   1   1      1    0    1   1   1
## 6    1   1   1   1   1      1    0    1   0   2
## 11   1   1   1   1   1      1    0    0   1   2
## 4    1   1   1   1   1      1    0    0   0   3
##      0   0   0   0   0      0   33   75  85 193
```

Additionally, we can assess the correlation:

1. Between variables with missing values

2. Between variables with missing values and variable with non-missing values
    ues

First, we need to take variables with missing values only. Then, we code a missing value with 1 and non-missing value with 0.

```
dummyNA <-
  as.data.frame(abs(is.na(coroNA))) %>%
  select(age, race, chol) # pick variable with missing values only
head(dummyNA)
```

```
##   age race chol
## 1   0    0    0
## 2   0    0    0
## 3   0    0    0
## 4   1    0    0
## 5   1    0    0
## 6   0    0    0
```

We assess the correlation between variables with missing values.

```
cor(dummyNA) %>% round(digits = 2)
```

```
##         age race  chol
## age    1.00 0.09 -0.11
## race   0.09 1.00  0.07
## chol  -0.11 0.07  1.00
```

There is no strong correlation between variables with missing values. We can conclude that the missing values in one variable is not related to the missing values in another variable.

The second correlation is between variables with missing values and variable with non-missing values. First, we need to change the categorical variable into a numeric value to get a correlation for all the variables.

```
cor(coroNA %>% mutate_if(is.factor, as.numeric),
    dummyNA, use = "pairwise.complete.obs") %>%
  round(digits = 2)
```

```
## Warning in cor(coroNA %>% mutate_if(is.factor, as.numeric), dummyNA, use =
## "pairwise.complete.obs"): the standard deviation is zero
```

```
##         age race chol
## age      NA 0.04 0.04
```

```
## race      0.02    NA  0.01
## chol     -0.11 -0.06    NA
## id        0.01 -0.06 -0.07
## cad       0.02  0.05 -0.17
## sbp      -0.07  0.04  0.17
## dbp      -0.04  0.04  0.17
## bmi       0.13 -0.08 -0.76
## gender    0.07  0.03 -0.07
```

We can safely ignore the warning generated in the result. Variables on the left side are variable with non-missing values and variables on the top of the columns are variables with missing values. There is a high correlation (-0.76) between bmi and chol, indicating values of chol are more likely to be missing at lower values of bmi.

Lastly, we can do a Little's test to determine if the missing data is MCAR or other types. The null hypothesis is the missing data is MCAR. Thus, a higher p value indicates probability of missing data is MCAR. The test shows that the missingness in our data is either MAR or MNAR.

```
mcar_test(coroNA)
```

```
## # A tibble: 1 x 4
##   statistic    df  p.value missing.patterns
##       <dbl> <dbl>    <dbl>            <int>
## 1      158.    51 8.25e-13                8
```

13.6   Handling Missing Data

We going to cover four approaches to handling missing data:

1. Listwise deletion
2. Simple imputation:
    - Mean substitution
    - Median substitution
    - Mode substitution
3. Single imputation:
    - Regression imputation
    - Stochastic regression imputation
    - Decision tree imputation
4. Multiple imputation

Each approach has their own caveats which we will cover in each section below.

13.6.1 Listwise deletion

Listwise or case deletion is the default setting in R. By default, R will exclude all the rows with missing data.

```
lw <- lm(dbp ~ ., data = coroNA)
summary(lw)
```

```
##
## Call:
## lm(formula = dbp ~ ., data = coroNA)
##
## Residuals:
##      Min       1Q   Median       3Q      Max
## -16.7770  -3.8094  -0.0874   3.5889  13.3479
##
## Coefficients:
##                 Estimate Std. Error t value Pr(>|t|)
## (Intercept)   34.6358468 20.5615343   1.684   0.0979 .
## age           -0.2764718  0.2139740  -1.292   0.2018
## raceindian     4.6080430  2.9423909   1.566   0.1232
## racemalay     -0.1318924  2.6075792  -0.051   0.9598
## chol           0.7174697  0.8142408   0.881   0.3821
## id             0.0000390  0.0006004   0.065   0.9484
## cadno cad     -1.2884879  2.2026942  -0.585   0.5610
## sbp            0.5390141  0.0502732  10.722 5.48e-15 ***
## bmi           -0.4189575  0.4086179  -1.025   0.3098
## genderwoman    2.3084961  1.6749082   1.378   0.1738
## ---
## Signif. codes:  0 '***' 0.001 '**' 0.01 '*' 0.05 '.' 0.1 ' ' 1
##
## Residual standard error: 6.218 on 54 degrees of freedom
##   (136 observations deleted due to missingness)
## Multiple R-squared:  0.7581, Adjusted R-squared:  0.7177
## F-statistic:  18.8 on 9 and 54 DF,  p-value: 1.05e-13
```

As shown in the information above (at the bottom), 136 rows or observations were excluded due to missingness. Listwise deletion approach able to produce an unbiased result only when the missing data is MCAR, and the amount of missing data is relatively small.

13.6.2 Simple imputation

A simple imputation includes mean, median and mode substitution is a relatively easy approach. In this approach, the missing values is replaced by a mean or median for numerical variable, and mode for categorical variable. This simple imputation approach only appropriate if missing data is MCAR and the amount of missing data is relatively small.

1. Mean substitution

replace_na will replace the missing values in age with its mean.

```
mean_sub <-
  coroNA %>%
  mutate(age = replace_na(age, mean(age, na.rm = T)))

summary(mean_sub)
```

```
##      age            race          chol            id              cad
## Min.   :33.00   chinese:31   Min.   :4.000   Min.   :   1.0   cad   : 37
## 1st Qu.:46.00   indian :45   1st Qu.:5.362   1st Qu.: 901.5   no cad:163
## Median :48.02   malay  :49   Median :6.050   Median :2243.5
## Mean   :48.02   NA's   :75   Mean   :6.114   Mean   :2218.3
## 3rd Qu.:49.00                3rd Qu.:6.875   3rd Qu.:3346.8
## Max.   :62.00                Max.   :9.350   Max.   :4696.0
##                              NA's   :33
##      sbp             dbp             bmi          gender
## Min.   : 88.0   Min.   : 56.00   Min.   :28.99   man   :100
## 1st Qu.:115.0   1st Qu.: 72.00   1st Qu.:36.10   woman :100
## Median :126.0   Median : 80.00   Median :37.80
## Mean   :130.2   Mean   : 82.31   Mean   :37.45
## 3rd Qu.:144.0   3rd Qu.: 92.00   3rd Qu.:39.20
## Max.   :187.0   Max.   :120.00   Max.   :45.03
##
```

2. Median substitution

replace_na will replace the missing values in age with its median.

```
med_sub <-
  coroNA %>%
  mutate(age = replace_na(age, median(age, na.rm = T)))

summary(med_sub)
```

```
##      age            race          chol            id              cad
## Min.   :33.00   chinese:31   Min.   :4.000   Min.   :   1.0   cad   : 37
```

```
## 1st Qu.:46.00    indian :45    1st Qu.:5.362    1st Qu.: 901.5    no cad:163
## Median :48.00    malay  :49    Median :6.050    Median :2243.5
## Mean   :48.01    NA's   :75    Mean   :6.114    Mean   :2218.3
## 3rd Qu.:49.00                  3rd Qu.:6.875    3rd Qu.:3346.8
## Max.   :62.00                  Max.   :9.350    Max.   :4696.0
##                                NA's   :33
##        sbp              dbp             bmi          gender
## Min.   : 88.0    Min.   : 56.00   Min.   :28.99   man   :100
## 1st Qu.:115.0    1st Qu.: 72.00   1st Qu.:36.10   woman:100
## Median :126.0    Median : 80.00   Median :37.80
## Mean   :130.2    Mean   : 82.31   Mean   :37.45
## 3rd Qu.:144.0    3rd Qu.: 92.00   3rd Qu.:39.20
## Max.   :187.0    Max.   :120.00   Max.   :45.03
##
```

3. Mode substitution

We need to find the mode, the most frequent level or group in the variable. In race variable, it is malay.

```
table(coroNA$race)
```

```
##
## chinese  indian   malay
##      31      45      49
```

replace_na will replace the missing values in race with its mode.

```
mode_sub <-
  coroNA %>%
  mutate(race = replace_na(race, "malay"))
```

```
summary(mode_sub)
```

```
##       age             race           chol             id              cad
## Min.   :33.00   chinese: 31   Min.   :4.000   Min.   :   1.0   cad   : 37
## 1st Qu.:43.00   indian : 45   1st Qu.:5.362   1st Qu.: 901.5   no cad:163
## Median :48.00   malay  :124   Median :6.050   Median :2243.5
## Mean   :48.02                 Mean   :6.114   Mean   :2218.3
## 3rd Qu.:53.00                 3rd Qu.:6.875   3rd Qu.:3346.8
## Max.   :62.00                 Max.   :9.350   Max.   :4696.0
## NA's   :85                    NA's   :33
##        sbp             dbp             bmi          gender
## Min.   : 88.0   Min.   : 56.00   Min.   :28.99   man   :100
```

```
## 1st Qu.:115.0    1st Qu.: 72.00    1st Qu.:36.10    woman:100
## Median :126.0    Median : 80.00    Median :37.80
## Mean   :130.2    Mean   : 82.31    Mean   :37.45
## 3rd Qu.:144.0    3rd Qu.: 92.00    3rd Qu.:39.20
## Max.   :187.0    Max.   :120.00    Max.   :45.03
##
```

13.6.3 Single imputation

In single imputation, missing data is imputed by any method producing a single set of a complete dataset. In fact, the simple imputation approaches (mean, median and mode) are part of single imputation techniques. Single imputation is better compared to the previous techniques that we have covered so far. This approach incorporate more information from other variables to impute the missing values. However, this approach produce a result with a small standard error, which reflect a false precision in the result. Additionally, a single imputation approach do not take into account uncertainty about the missing data (except for stochastic regression imputation). Additionally, this approach is applicable if the missing data is at least MAR.

1. Regression imputation

We will do a linear regression imputation for numerical variables (age and chol) and multinomial or polytomous logistic regression for categorical variable (since race has three levels: Malay, Chinese and Indian).

We run `mice()` with `maxit = 0` (zero iteration) to get a model specification and further removed id variable as it is not useful for the analysis. Here, we do not actually run the imputation yet as the iteration is zero (`maxit = 0`).

```
ini <- mice(coroNA %>% select(-id), m = 1, maxit = 0)
ini
```

```
## Class: mids
## Number of multiple imputations:  1
## Imputation methods:
##         age       race       chol        cad        sbp        dbp        bmi     gender
##       "pmm"  "polyreg"      "pmm"         ""         ""         ""         ""         ""
## PredictorMatrix:
##        age race chol cad sbp dbp bmi gender
## age      0    1    1   1   1   1   1      1
## race     1    0    1   1   1   1   1      1
## chol     1    1    0   1   1   1   1      1
## cad      1    1    1   0   1   1   1      1
## sbp      1    1    1   1   0   1   1      1
## dbp      1    1    1   1   1   0   1      1
```

By default, `mice()` use predictive mean matching (pmm) for a numerical variable, binary logistic regression (logreg) for a categorical variable with two levels and multinomial or polytomous logistic regression (polyreg) for a categorical variable with more than two level. `mice()` will not assign any method for variable with non-missing values by default (denote by " " in the section of imputation method above).

We going to change the method for numerical variable (age and chol) to a linear regression.

```
meth <- ini$method
meth[c(1,3)] <- "norm.predict"
meth
```

```
##                age            race           chol          cad          sbp
## "norm.predict"       "polyreg" "norm.predict"          ""           ""
##                dbp            bmi         gender
##                 ""             ""             ""
```

`mice()` function contains a few arguments:

- `m`: number of imputed sets (will be used in the multiple imputation later)
- `method`: to specify a method of imputation
- `predictorMatrix`: to specify predictors for imputation
- `printFlag`: print history on the R console
- `seed`: random number for reproducibility

```
regImp <- mice(coroNA %>% select(-id),
               m = 1, method = meth, printFlag = F, seed = 123)
regImp
```

```
## Class: mids
## Number of multiple imputations:  1
## Imputation methods:
##                age            race           chol          cad          sbp
## "norm.predict"       "polyreg" "norm.predict"          ""           ""
##                dbp            bmi         gender
##                 ""             ""             ""
## PredictorMatrix:
##        age race chol cad sbp dbp bmi gender
## age      0    1    1   1   1   1   1      1
## race     1    0    1   1   1   1   1      1
## chol     1    1    0   1   1   1   1      1
## cad      1    1    1   0   1   1   1      1
## sbp      1    1    1   1   0   1   1      1
## dbp      1    1    1   1   1   0   1      1
```

Here, we can see the summary of our imputation model:

1. Number of multiple imputation
2. Imputation methods
3. PredictorMatrix

We can further assess the full predictor matrix from the model.

```
regImp$predictorMatrix
```

```
##           age race chol cad sbp dbp bmi gender
## age         0    1    1   1   1   1   1      1
## race        1    0    1   1   1   1   1      1
## chol        1    1    0   1   1   1   1      1
## cad         1    1    1   0   1   1   1      1
## sbp         1    1    1   1   0   1   1      1
## dbp         1    1    1   1   1   0   1      1
## bmi         1    1    1   1   1   1   0      1
## gender      1    1    1   1   1   1   1      0
```

The predictor matrix denotes the variable to be imputed at the left side and the predictors at the top of the column. 1 indicates a predictor while 0 zero indicates a non-predictor. This predictor matrix can be changed accordingly if needed by changing 1 to 0 (a predictor to a non-predictor) or vise versa. Noted that the diagonal is 0 as the variable is not allowed to impute itself.

As an example, to impute missing values in age, all of the variables are used as predictors except for age itself as shown in the predictor matrix. So, the outcome variable ($\hat{y}$) in linear regression equation will be the imputed variable.

$$\hat{y} = \beta_0 + \beta_1 x_1 + \beta_2 x_2 + \ldots + \beta_k x_k$$

So, the above equation for imputed age variable in the first row of the predictor matrix will be:

$$age = \beta_0 + \beta_1(race) + \beta_2(chol) + \beta_3(cad) + \beta_4(sbp) + \beta_5(dbp) + \beta_6(bmi) + \beta_6(gender)$$

Although it seems that we impute all the missing values in each variable simultaneously, in actuality each imputation model will run separately. So, in our data, on top of the imputation model for age, we have another imputation models for race and chol variables. Fortunately, we do not have to concern much about which variable to be used as a predictor as `mice()` will automatically select the useful predictors for each variables with missing values. Further information on how `mice` do this automatic selection can assessed by typing `quickpred()` in the RStudio console.

We can asses the imputed dataset as follows:

```
coro_regImp <- complete(regImp, 1)
summary(coro_regImp)
```

```
##       age            race         chol            cad           sbp
## Min.   :33.00   chinese:56   Min.   :4.000   cad   : 37   Min.   : 88.0
## 1st Qu.:41.32   indian :67   1st Qu.:5.445   no cad:163   1st Qu.:115.0
## Median :47.00   malay  :77   Median :6.092                Median :126.0
## Mean   :47.68                Mean   :6.144                Mean   :130.2
## 3rd Qu.:53.38                3rd Qu.:6.774                3rd Qu.:144.0
## Max.   :62.00                Max.   :9.350                Max.   :187.0
##       dbp            bmi           gender
## Min.   : 56.00   Min.   :28.99   man   :100
## 1st Qu.: 72.00   1st Qu.:36.10   woman:100
## Median : 80.00   Median :37.80
## Mean   : 82.31   Mean   :37.45
## 3rd Qu.: 92.00   3rd Qu.:39.20
## Max.   :120.00   Max.   :45.03
```

2. Stochastic regression imputation

Stochastic regression imputation is an extension of regression imputation. This method attempts to account for the missing data uncertainty by adding a noise or extra variance. This method only applicable for numerical variable.

First, we get a model specification.

```
ini <- mice(coroNA %>% select(-id), m = 1, maxit = 0)
ini
```

```
## Class: mids
## Number of multiple imputations:  1
## Imputation methods:
##       age      race      chol       cad       sbp       dbp       bmi    gender
##     "pmm" "polyreg"     "pmm"        ""        ""        ""        ""        ""
## PredictorMatrix:
##        age race chol cad sbp dbp bmi gender
## age      0    1    1   1   1   1   1      1
## race     1    0    1   1   1   1   1      1
## chol     1    1    0   1   1   1   1      1
## cad      1    1    1   0   1   1   1      1
## sbp      1    1    1   1   0   1   1      1
## dbp      1    1    1   1   1   0   1      1
```

Then, we specify the imputation method to stochastic regression (norm.nob) for all numerical variables with missing values (age and chol).

```
meth <- ini$method
meth[c(1,3)] <- "norm.nob"
meth
```

```
##        age        race        chol        cad        sbp        dbp        bmi
## "norm.nob"  "polyreg"  "norm.nob"         ""         ""         ""         ""
##      gender
##          ""
```

Then, we run mice().

```
srImp <- mice(coroNA %>% select(-id),
              m = 1, method = meth, printFlag = F, seed = 123)
srImp
```

```
## Class: mids
## Number of multiple imputations:  1
## Imputation methods:
##        age        race        chol        cad        sbp        dbp        bmi
## "norm.nob"  "polyreg"  "norm.nob"         ""         ""         ""         ""
##      gender
##          ""
## PredictorMatrix:
##        age race chol cad sbp dbp bmi gender
## age      0    1    1   1   1   1   1      1
## race     1    0    1   1   1   1   1      1
## chol     1    1    0   1   1   1   1      1
## cad      1    1    1   0   1   1   1      1
## sbp      1    1    1   1   0   1   1      1
## dbp      1    1    1   1   1   0   1      1
```

Here is the imputed dataset.

```
coro_srImp <- complete(srImp, 1)
summary(coro_srImp)
```

```
##       age            race          chol            cad           sbp
## Min.   :31.54   chinese:52   Min.   :4.000   cad   : 37   Min.   : 88.0
## 1st Qu.:42.16   indian :70   1st Qu.:5.390   no cad:163   1st Qu.:115.0
## Median :46.70   malay  :78   Median :6.105                Median :126.0
## Mean   :47.46                Mean   :6.219                Mean   :130.2
```

```
##   3rd Qu.:52.25              3rd Qu.:7.005          3rd Qu.:144.0
##   Max.   :66.41              Max.   :9.600          Max.   :187.0
##        dbp              bmi            gender
##   Min.   : 56.00   Min.   :28.99   man  :100
##   1st Qu.: 72.00   1st Qu.:36.10   woman:100
##   Median : 80.00   Median :37.80
##   Mean   : 82.31   Mean   :37.45
##   3rd Qu.: 92.00   3rd Qu.:39.20
##   Max.   :120.00   Max.   :45.03
```

3. Decision tree imputation

Decision tree or classification and regression tree (CART) is a popular method in machine learning area. This method can be applied to impute a missing values for both numerical and categorical variables.

First, we get a model specification.

```
ini <- mice(coroNA %>% select(-id), m = 1, maxit = 0)
ini
```

```
## Class: mids
## Number of multiple imputations:  1
## Imputation methods:
##         age        race        chol         cad         sbp         dbp         bmi      gender
##      "pmm"   "polyreg"       "pmm"          ""          ""          ""          ""          ""
## PredictorMatrix:
##         age race chol cad sbp dbp bmi gender
## age       0    1    1   1   1   1   1      1
## race      1    0    1   1   1   1   1      1
## chol      1    1    0   1   1   1   1      1
## cad       1    1    1   0   1   1   1      1
## sbp       1    1    1   1   0   1   1      1
## dbp       1    1    1   1   1   0   1      1
```

Then, we specify the imputation methods for all variable with missing values (age, race and chol) to decision tree.

```
meth <- ini$method
meth[1:3] <- "cart"
meth
```

```
##      age    race    chol     cad     sbp     dbp     bmi gender
##   "cart"  "cart"  "cart"      ""      ""      ""      ""     ""
```

Next, we run the imputation model.

```
cartImp <- mice(coroNA %>% select(-id),
                m = 1, method = meth, printFlag = F, seed = 123)
cartImp
```

```
## Class: mids
## Number of multiple imputations:  1
## Imputation methods:
##    age   race   chol    cad    sbp    dbp    bmi gender
## "cart" "cart" "cart"     ""     ""     ""     ""     ""
## PredictorMatrix:
##        age race chol cad sbp dbp bmi gender
## age      0    1    1   1   1   1   1      1
## race     1    0    1   1   1   1   1      1
## chol     1    1    0   1   1   1   1      1
## cad      1    1    1   0   1   1   1      1
## sbp      1    1    1   1   0   1   1      1
## dbp      1    1    1   1   1   0   1      1
```

Here is the imputed dataset.

```
coro_cartImp <- complete(cartImp, 1)
summary(coro_cartImp)
```

```
##       age            race          chol            cad           sbp
## Min.   :33.00   chinese:56   Min.   :4.000   cad   : 37   Min.   : 88.0
## 1st Qu.:42.50   indian :70   1st Qu.:5.390   no cad:163   1st Qu.:115.0
## Median :47.00   malay  :74   Median :6.050                Median :126.0
## Mean   :47.92                Mean   :6.085                Mean   :130.2
## 3rd Qu.:53.00                3rd Qu.:6.765                3rd Qu.:144.0
## Max.   :62.00                Max.   :9.350                Max.   :187.0
##       dbp             bmi           gender
## Min.   : 56.00   Min.   :28.99   man   :100
## 1st Qu.: 72.00   1st Qu.:36.10   woman :100
## Median : 80.00   Median :37.80
## Mean   : 82.31   Mean   :37.45
## 3rd Qu.: 92.00   3rd Qu.:39.20
## Max.   :120.00   Max.   :45.03
```

13.6.4   Multiple imputation

Multiple imputation is an advanced approach to missing data. In this approach, several imputed datasets will be generated. Analyses will be run on each imputed datasets. Then, all the results will be combined into a pooled result. The advantage of multiple imputation is this approach takes into account uncertainty regarding the missing data, by which the single imputation approach may fail to do. Generally, this approach is applicable if the missing data is at least MAR.

Flow of the multiple imputation is quite similar to the single imputation since we are using the same package. The number of imputed set, m by default is set to 5 in `mice()`. In general, the higher number of m is better, though this makes the computation longer. For moderate amount of missing data, m between 5 to 20 should be enough. Another recommendation is to set m to the average percentage of missing data. However, for this example we going to run the default values.

```
miImp <- mice(coroNA %>% select(-id), m = 5, printFlag = F, seed = 123)
miImp
```

```
## Class: mids
## Number of multiple imputations:  5
## Imputation methods:
##       age     race     chol      cad      sbp      dbp      bmi   gender
##     "pmm" "polyreg"    "pmm"       ""       ""       ""       ""       ""
## PredictorMatrix:
##        age race chol cad sbp dbp bmi gender
## age      0    1    1   1   1   1   1      1
## race     1    0    1   1   1   1   1      1
## chol     1    1    0   1   1   1   1      1
## cad      1    1    1   0   1   1   1      1
## sbp      1    1    1   1   0   1   1      1
## dbp      1    1    1   1   1   0   1      1
```

We can see in the result, the number of imputations is 5. We can extract the first imputation set as follows:

```
complete(miImp, 1) %>%
  summary()
```

```
##       age            race          chol            cad            sbp
##  Min.   :33.00   chinese:50   Min.   :4.000   cad    : 37   Min.   : 88.0
##  1st Qu.:43.00   indian :72   1st Qu.:5.170   no cad:163   1st Qu.:115.0
##  Median :48.00   malay  :78   Median :5.968                Median :126.0
##  Mean   :47.94                Mean   :5.993                Mean   :130.2
##  3rd Qu.:53.00                3rd Qu.:6.703                3rd Qu.:144.0
##  Max.   :62.00                Max.   :9.350                Max.   :187.0
##       dbp             bmi          gender
##  Min.   : 56.00   Min.   :28.99   man  :100
##  1st Qu.: 72.00   1st Qu.:36.10   woman:100
```

```
##   Median : 80.00   Median :37.80
##   Mean   : 82.31   Mean   :37.45
##   3rd Qu.: 92.00   3rd Qu.:39.20
##   Max.   :120.00   Max.   :45.03
```

Next, we need to check for convergence of the algorithm.

```
plot(miImp)
```

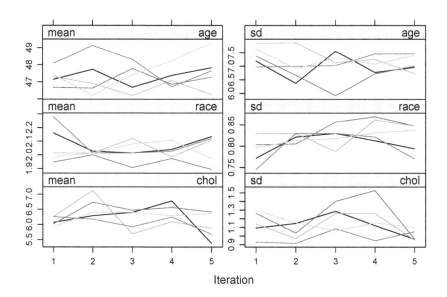

The line in the plot should be intermingled and free of any trend. The number of iteration can be further increased to make sure of this.

```
miImp2 <- mice.mids(miImp, maxit = 35, printFlag = F)
plot(miImp2)
```

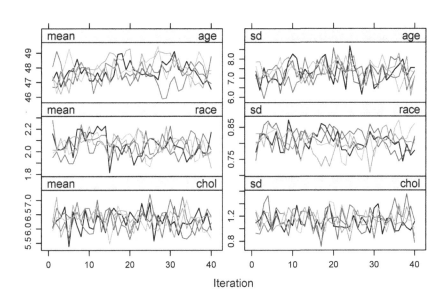

Once the imputed datasets are obtained, an analysis (for example, a linear regression) can be run as follows:

```
lr_mi <- with(miImp, glm(dbp ~ age + race + chol + cad + sbp + bmi + gender))
pool(lr_mi) %>%
  summary(conf.int = T)
```

```
##              term     estimate    std.error    statistic          df      p.value
## 1 (Intercept) 25.85805530 13.21741793  1.95636209  34.41840 5.857610e-02
## 2         age -0.09649575  0.21229624 -0.45453348  10.34947 6.588297e-01
## 3   raceindian -0.07034050  2.57995900 -0.02726419  12.32421 9.786855e-01
## 4    racemalay  0.20029789  1.68514315  0.11886105  59.44295 9.057862e-01
## 5        chol  1.33244955  0.52966992  2.51562245  89.92925 1.365737e-02
## 6    cadno cad -1.43834422  1.43322822 -1.00356956 160.05725 3.171009e-01
## 7         sbp  0.51358079  0.03015353 17.03219634 186.95165 6.967240e-40
## 8         bmi -0.35959227  0.20258274 -1.77503907 136.19191 7.812525e-02
## 9 genderwoman  1.30467626  1.04972267  1.24287709 185.09416 2.154853e-01
##       2.5 %      97.5 %
## 1 -0.9909476 52.70705817
## 2 -0.5673651  0.37437357
## 3 -5.6752310  5.53454998
## 4 -3.1711401  3.57173588
## 5  0.2801565  2.38474258
```

```
## 6 -4.2688212  1.39213272
## 7  0.4540959  0.57306569
## 8 -0.7602069  0.04102233
## 9 -0.7662831  3.37563562
```

We can use `mutate_if()` from `dplyr` package to round up the numbers to two decimal points.

```
pool(lr_mi) %>%
  summary(conf.int = T) %>%
  as.data.frame() %>%
  mutate_if(is.numeric, round, 2)
```

```
##               term estimate std.error statistic     df p.value  2.5 % 97.5 %
## 1 (Intercept)    25.86     13.22      1.96  34.42    0.06  -0.99  52.71
## 2         age    -0.10      0.21     -0.45  10.35    0.66  -0.57   0.37
## 3   raceindian   -0.07      2.58     -0.03  12.32    0.98  -5.68   5.53
## 4    racemalay    0.20      1.69      0.12  59.44    0.91  -3.17   3.57
## 5        chol     1.33      0.53      2.52  89.93    0.01   0.28   2.38
## 6     cadno cad  -1.44      1.43     -1.00 160.06    0.32  -4.27   1.39
## 7         sbp     0.51      0.03     17.03 186.95    0.00   0.45   0.57
## 8         bmi    -0.36      0.20     -1.78 136.19    0.08  -0.76   0.04
## 9 genderwoman    1.30      1.05      1.24 185.09    0.22  -0.77   3.38
```

`mice` package has provided an easy flow to run the analysis for multiple imputation:

1. `mice()`: impute the missing data
2. `with()`: run a statistical analysis
3. `pool()`: pool the results

Additionally, a model comparison can be done as well. There are three methods available for the model comparison:

1. `D1()`: multivariate Wald test
2. `D2()`: pools test statistics from each analysis of the imputed datasets
3. `D3()`: likelihood-ratio test statistics

`D2()` is less powerful compared to the other two methods.

```
lr_mi2 <- with(miImp, glm(dbp ~ race + chol + cad + sbp + bmi + gender))
summary(D1(lr_mi, lr_mi2))
```

```
##
## Models:
```

```
## model                                           formula
##     1 dbp ~ age + race + chol + cad + sbp + bmi + gender
##     2       dbp ~ race + chol + cad + sbp + bmi + gender
##
## Comparisons:
##   test statistic df1 df2 dfcom   p.value      riv
## 1 ~~ 2 0.2066007   1   4   191 0.6730188 1.379672
##
## Number of imputations:  5   Method D1
```

Multivariate Wald test is not significant. Hence, removing age from the model does not reduce its predictive power. We can safely exclude age variable to aim for a parsimonious model.

```
summary(D2(lr_mi, lr_mi2))
```

```
##
## Models:
##   model                                         formula
##     1 dbp ~ age + race + chol + cad + sbp + bmi + gender
##     2       dbp ~ race + chol + cad + sbp + bmi + gender
##
## Comparisons:
##   test     statistic df1     df2 dfcom p.value      riv
## 1 ~~ 2 -0.002254427   1 16.1953    NA       1 0.9879772
##
## Number of imputations:  5   Method D2 (wald)
```

```
summary(D3(lr_mi, lr_mi2))
```

```
##
## Models:
##   model                                           formula
##     1 dbp ~ age + race + chol + cad + sbp + bmi + gender
##     2       dbp ~ race + chol + cad + sbp + bmi + gender
##
## Comparisons:
##   test statistic df1     df2 dfcom   p.value      riv
## 1 ~~ 2 0.1946719   1 10.83101   191 0.6677344 1.549127
##
## Number of imputations:  5   Method D3
```

Also, we get a similar result from the remaining two methods for the model comparison. However, this may not always be the case. Generally, D1() and D3() are preferred and equally good for a sample size more than 200. However, for a small sample size (n < 200), D1() is better. Besides, D2() should be used with cautious, especially in large datasets with many missing values as it may produce a false positive estimate.

13.7   Presentation

gtsummary package can be used for all the analyses run on the approaches of handling missing data that we have covered in this chapter. Here is an example to get a nice table using tbl_regression() from a linear regression model run on the multiple imputation approach.

```
tbl_regression(lr_mi2)
```

Characteristic	Beta	95% CI	p-value
race			
chinese	—	—	
indian	−0.86	−4.1, 2.3	0.6
malay	0.73	−2.0, 3.5	0.6
chol	1.3	0.29, 2.3	0.012
cad			
cad	—	—	
no cad	−1.3	−4.0, 1.5	0.4
sbp	0.51	0.45, 0.57	< 0.001
bmi	−0.36	−0.77, 0.04	0.076
gender			
man	—	—	
woman	1.4	−0.67, 3.4	0.2

13.8   Resources

We suggest Schafer and Graham (2002) and Kang (2013) for theoretical details on the missing data, Zhang (2015) for missing data exploration and Martin W Heymans (2019) and van Buuren (2018) for more details on single and multiple imputation.

13.9 Summary

This chapter provides an overview of the type of missing data and how to investigate it, either visually, descriptively or statistically. This chapter also covers practical methods for handling missing data in research from a simple method like a listwise deletion to a more advanced method of multiple imputation. There is extensive literature on the approach to missing data that are not included in this brief chapter. However, we hope this chapter will give readers a solid starting point to further explore other resources.

14

Model Building and Variable Selection

14.1 Objectives

At the end of the chapter, readers will be able to:

- understand basic concept of univariable and multivariable analysis
- know about some workflows or methods multivariable model building
- compare different types of variables selection

14.2 Introduction

In previous chapters, we avoided going into details of model building and variable selection processes. This is because the choices, workflows and approaches for both processes varies and depends on the objectives and preferences of the users or analysts. It is very rare that a statistical model has a single independent variable or predictor only. Almost always, the models contain more than one single independent variable. The collection of independent variables can consist of numerical only or categorical only or a mix of numerical and categorical independent variables.

Statisticians coin the model with one independent variable as a univariate model and a model with more than one independent variables as multivariate model but some analysts prefer to call these as *univariable* and multivariable model. Stata (2022a) claimed that *multivariable* is mostly biostatistical in usage. It does not mean something other than *multivariate*. He added that univariate, bivariate, multivariate just count the number of variables, one, two or many.

variate means random variable in statistics terminology. If we literally follow the definition, *multivariate analysis* may only cover non-regression type analyses for multiple random variables (e.g. principal component analysis and factor analysis) or regression analyses with multiple outcome variables (e.g. multivariate analysis of variance). However, in most situations described as "multivariate analysis", medical researchers' intentions are clear: adjust for multiple covariates as explanatory variables in regression models. In fact, we usually model the conditional expectation $E(Y|X)$ by regression analysis in observational studies where the joint distribution

(X, Y) is not controlled by researchers. We thus believe that *multivariate adjustment* or *multivariate analysis* is not necessarily misuse of the terminology as stated by others (Peters, 2008).

14.3   Model Building

The main goal of a statistical analysis of effects should be the production of the most accurate (valid and precise) effect estimates obtainable from the data and available software (Greenland et al., 2016). Usually there are three model-building strategies according to Hafermann et al. (2021) and Greenland and Pearce (2015) :

- Adjust all: Enter all the potential confounders in the model (only one set of covariates is considered, although the form of the model may be varied).
- Predictor selection: Select covariates on the basis of some measure of their ability to predict outcome or exposure (or both) given other covariates in the model.
- Change in estimate (CIE) selection: Select covariates on the basis of the change in the exposure effect estimate upon excluding them, given the other covariates in the model.

Prerequisites for model buildings include (Greenland et al., 2016):

- carefully completed data checking, data description and data summarization
- all quantitative variables have been: re-centered to ensure that zero is a meaningful reference value present in the data;
- all quantitative variables have been rescaled so that their units are meaningful differences within the range of the data;
- univariate distributions and background (contextual) information have been used to select categories or an appropriately flexible form (e.g. splines) for detailed modeling

Greenland et al. (2016) advised that controlling too many variables can lead to or aggravate problems arising from data sparsity or from high multiple correlation of exposure with the controlled confounders (which we term multicollinearity). They reminded not to control for intermediates (variables on the causal pathway between exposure and diseases) and their descendants. Also not to control for variables that are not part of minimal sufficient adjustment sets, whose control may increase bias.

If background knowledge is only based on a few preceding studies without sufficient biological support, the methodology of these studies should be carefully investigated, and uncertainties related to the selection or non-selection of variables in such studies should be critically inferred (Hafermann et al., 2021). The covariates may be forced variables, which we always want to control (typically for age and sex), or unforced variables for which the decision to control may be data based (Greenland and Pearce, 2015).

It is not recommended to adjust for every available Covariate because it has some practical drawbacks. The set of covariates it identifies can be far larger than needed for adequate confounding control (far from minimally sufficient) and may be clumsy for subsequent analyses. there may be many covariates whose causal status (and thus their fulfillment of the criterion) is uncertain. Controlling too many variables by conventional means can lead to or aggravate two closely related problems: (a) data sparsity, in which full control results in too few subjects at crucial combinations of the variables, with consequent inflation of estimates, and (b) multicollinearity, by which we mean high multiple correlation (or more generally, high association) of the controlled variables with study exposures (Greenland and Pearce, 2015).

14.4   Variable Selection for Prediction

Variable selection means choosing among many variables which to include in a particular model, that is, to select appropriate variables from a complete list of variables by removing those that are irrelevant or redundant. The purpose of such selection is to determine a set of variables that will provide the best fit for the model so that accurate predictions can be made (Chowdhury and Turin, 2020).

Chowdhury and Turin (2020) listed some variable selection methods:

- Backward elimination
- Forward selection
- Stepwise selection
- All possible subset selection

14.4.1   Backward elimination

Backward elimination is the simplest of all variable selection methods. This method starts with a full model that considers all of the variables to be included in the model. Variables then are deleted one by one from the full model until all remaining variables are considered to have some significant contribution to the outcome. The variable with the smallest test statistic (a measure of the variable's contribution to the model) less than the cut-off value or with the highest p value greater than the cut-off value—the least significant variable—is deleted first. Then the model is refitted without the deleted variable and the test statistics or p values are recomputed. Again, the variable with the smallest test statistic or with the highest p value greater than the cut-off value is deleted in the refitted model. This process is repeated until every remaining variable is significant at the cut-off value. The cut-off value associated with the p value is sometimes referred to as 'p-to-remove' and does not have to be set at 0.05.

14.4.2   Forward selection

The forward selection method of variable selection is the reverse of the backward elimination method. The method starts with no variables in the model and then adds variables to the model one by one until any variable not included in the model can add any significant contribution to the outcome of the model.1 At each step, each variable excluded from the model is tested for inclusion in the model. If an excluded variable is added to the model, the test statistic or p value is calculated. The variable with the largest test statistic greater than the cut-off value or the lowest p value less than the cut-off value is selected and added to the model. In other words, the most significant variable is added first. The model then is refitted with this variable and test statistics or p values are recomputed for all remaining variables. Again, the variable with the largest test statistic greater than the cut-off value or the lowest p value less than the cut-off value is chosen from among the remaining variables and added to the model. This process continues until no remaining variable is significant at the cut-off level when added to the model. In forward selection, if a variable is added to the model, it remains there.

14.4.3   Stepwise selection

Stepwise selection methods are a widely used variable selection technique, particularly in medical applications. This method is a combination of forward and backward selection procedures that allow moving in both directions, adding and removing variables at different steps. The process can start with both a backward elimination and forward selection approach. For example, if stepwise selection starts with forward selection, variables are added to the model one at a time based on statistical significance. At each step, after a variable is added, the procedure checks all the variables already added to the model to delete any variable that is not significant in the model. The process continues until every variable in the model is significant and every excluded variable is insignificant. Due to its similarity, this approach is sometimes considered as a modified forward selection.

14.4.4   All possible subset selection

In all possible subset selection, every possible combination of variables is checked to determine the best subset of variables for the prediction model. With this procedure, all one-variable, two-variable, three-variable models, and so on, are built to determine which one is the best according to some specific criteria. If there are K variables, then there are 2K possible models that can be built.

14.5 Stopping Rule and Selection Criteria in Automatic Variable Selection

In all stepwise selection methods including all subset selection, a stopping rule or selection criteria for inclusion or exclusion of variables need to be set. Generally, a standard significance level for hypothesis testing is used.7 However, other criteria are also frequently used as a stopping rule such as the AIC, BIC or Mallows' Cp statistic (Chowdhury and Turin, 2020).

14.6 Problems with Automatic Variable Selections

The problems with automatic variables selection include (Stata, 2022b):

- It yields R-squared values that are badly biased to be high.
- The F and chi-squared tests quoted next to each variable on the printout do not have the claimed distribution.
- The method yields confidence intervals for effects and predicted values that are falsely narrow
- It yields p-values that do not have the proper meaning, and the proper correction for them is a difficult problem.
- It gives biased regression coefficients that need shrinkage
- It has severe problems in the presence of collinearity.
- It is based on methods (e.g. F tests for nested models) that were intended to be used to test prespecified hypotheses.
- Increasing the sample size does not help very much
- It allows us to not think about the problem.
- It uses a lot of paper.

It addition to that, it is possible that automatic variable selection for example,

- stepwise methods will not necessarily produce the best model if there are redundant predictors (common problem).
- all-possible-subset methods produce the best model for each possible number of terms, but larger models need not necessarily be subsets of smaller ones, causing serious conceptual problems about the underlying logic of the investigation.

Models built from automatic variable selection may have an inflated risk of capitalizing on chance features of the data. They often fail when applied to new datasets. They are rarely tested in this way. And since the interpretation of coefficients in a model depends on the other terms included, *it seems unwise, to let an automatic algorithm determine the questions we do and do not ask about our data.*

14.7   Purposeful Variable Selection

Purposeful variable selection is proposed by Hosmer et al. (2013). In purposeful variable selection, the steps include

- Univariable analysis: Usually the variables that achieve statistical significance at p-value of 0.20 or known clinically important variables will go to the next steps.
- multivariable model comparison: This step fits the multivariable model comprising all variables identified in step one. Variables that do not contribute to the model (e.g. with a p value greater than traditional significance level) should be eliminated and a new smaller mode fits. These two models are then compared by using partial likelihood ratio test to make sure that the parsimonious model fits as well as the original model.
- linearity assumption for categorical outcome: In the step, continuous variables are checked for their linearity in relation to the logit of the outcome.
- checking interaction: An interaction between two variables implies that the effect of one variable on response variable is dependent on another variable.
- model checking

14.8   Summary

Model building and variable selection are two important processes in order to build an acceptable model for analysis. Parsimony and goodness-of-fit are inappropriate end goals for modeling, as indicated by simulation studies in which full-model analysis sometimes outperforms conventional selection strategies. The simple strategies include controlling of all potential confounders and eliminating some or all variables whose inclusion is of uncertain value. However, no methodology is foolproof and that modeling methods should be documented in enough detail so that readers can interpret results in light of the strengths and weaknesses of those methods.

Bibliography

Chang, W. (2013). *R Graphics Cookbook*. Oreilly and Associate Series. O'Reilly Media, Incorporated.

Chowdhury, M. Z. I. and Turin, T. C. (2020). Variable selection strategies and its importance in clinical prediction modelling. *Family Medicine and Community Health*, 8(1):e000262.

Daniel, W. and Cross, C. (2014). *Biostatistics: Basic Concepts and Methodology for the Health Sciences*. Wiley Series in Probability and Statistics Series. Wiley.

Doll, R. (1971). The age distribution of cancer: Implications for models of carcinogenesis. *Journal of the Royal Statistical Society. Series A (General)*, 134(2):133–155.

Everitt, B. S. and Hothorn, T. (2017). *HSAUR: A Handbook of Statistical Analyses Using R, First Edition*. R package version 1.3-9.

Fleiss, J. L., Levin, B., and Paik, M. C. (2003). *Statistical Methods for Rates and Proportions, Third Edition*. USA: John Wiley & Sons.

Frome, E. L. (1983). The analysis of rates using poisson regression models. *Biometrics*, 39(3):665–674.

Greenland, S., Daniel, R., and Pearce, N. (2016). Outcome modelling strategies in epidemiology: Traditional methods and basic alternatives. *International Journal of Epidemiology*, 45(2):565–575.

Greenland, S. and Pearce, N. (2015). Statistical foundations for model-based adjustments. *Annual Review of Public Health*, 36(1):89–108. PMID: 25785886.

Hafermann, L., Becher, H., Herrmann, C., Klein, N., Heinze, G., and Rauch, G. (2021). Statistical model building: Background "knowledge" based on inappropriate preselection causes misspecification. *BMC Medical Research Methodology*, 21:1–12.

Hosmer, D., Lemeshow, S., and Sturdivant, R. (2013). *Applied Logistic Regression*. Wiley Series in Probability and Statistics. Wiley.

Hu, S. (2007). Akaike information criterion. *Center for Research in Scientific Computation*, 93.

Kang, H. (2013). The prevention and handling of the missing data. *Korean Journal of Anesthesiology*, 64(5):402.

Kleinbaum, D. (2010). *Logistic Regression : A Self-learning Text*. Springer, New York.

Kleinbaum, D. G. and Klein, M. (2005). *Survival Analysis: A Self-Learning Text*. Springer Science and Business Media, LLC, New.

Lemeshow, S., May, S., and Hosmer Jr., D. W. (2008). *Applied Survival Analysis: Regression Modeling of Time-to-Event Data*. Wiley-Interscience, hardcover edition.

Long, J. and Freese, J. (2006). *Regression Models for Categorical Dependent Variables Using Stata, Second Edition*. A Stata Press publication. Taylor & Francis.

Martin W Heymans, I. E. (2019). *Applied Missing Data Analysis With SPSS and (R)Studio*. https://bookdown.org/mwheymans/bookmi/.

Neter, J., Kutner, M., Wasserman, M., and Nachtsheim, C. (2013). *Applied Linear Statistical Models, Fifth Edition (Pb 2013)*. Mc Graw Hill India, paperback edition.

Peters, T. J. (2008). Multifarious terminology: multivariable or multivariate? univariable or univariate? *Paediatric and Perinatal Epidemiology*, 22(6):506–506.

Schafer, J. L. and Graham, J. W. (2002). Missing data: Our view of the state of the art. *Psychological Methods*, 7(2):147–177.

Sjoberg, D. D., Whiting, K., Curry, M., Lavery, J. A., and Larmarange, J. (2021). Reproducible summary tables with the gtsummary package. *The R Journal*, 13:570–580.

Stata (2022a). Re: st: Proper usage: Univariate, bivariate, multivariate, multivariab. https://www.stata.com/statalist/archive/2013-10/msg00531.html. [Online; accessed 11 Nov 2022].

Stata (2022b). Stata faq: Problems with stepwise regression. https://www.stata.com/support/faqs/statistics/stepwise-regression-problems/. [Online; accessed 07 Nov 2022].

van Buuren, S. (2018). *Flexible Imputation of Missing Data, Second Edition*. Chapman and Hall/CRC.

Wickham, H., Chang, W., Henry, L., Pedersen, T. L., Takahashi, K., Wilke, C., Woo, K., Yutani, H., and Dunnington, D. (2020). *ggplot2: Create Elegant Data Visualisations Using the Grammar of Graphics*. R package version 3.3.2.

Wickham, H. and Grolemund, G. (2017). *R for Data Science: Import, Tidy, Transform, Visualize, and Model Data*. O'Reilly Media.

Wikipedia (2022). Akaike information criterion, wikipedia. the free encyclopedia. https://en.wikipedia.org/wiki/Akaike_information_criterion. [Online; accessed 07 Mar 2022].

Woodward, M. (2013). *Epidemiology: Study Design and Data Analysis, Third Edition*. Chapman & Hall/CRC Texts in Statistical Science. CRC Press.

Zhang, Z. (2015). Missing data exploration: Highlighting graphical presentation of missing pattern. *Annals of Translational Medicine*, 3:356.

Index

Printed in the United States
by Baker & Taylor Publisher Services